At Sara's Table
Chester Creek Cafe
20th Anniversary Cookbook

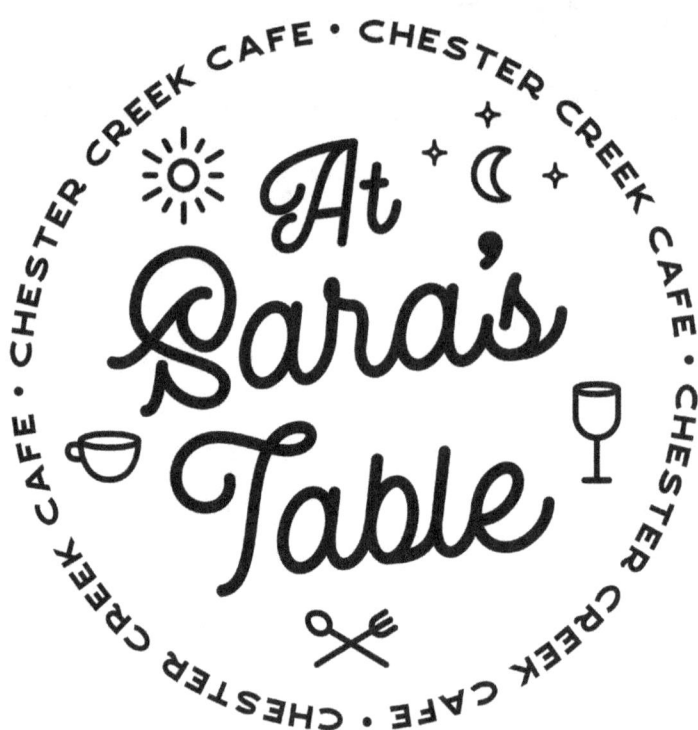

At Sara's Table

CHESTER CREEK CAFE • CHESTER CREEK CAFE • CHESTER CREEK CAFE • CHESTER CREEK CAFE • CHESTER CREEK CAFE •

At Sara's Table Chester Creek Cafe
20th Anniversary Cookbook

A celebration of the food, the farmers, the talent, and the vision that created this much-treasured Duluth restaurant.

Jillian Forte

ISBN: 9798987052303

Library of Congress Control Number is available on file.

Front cover image by Melissa Wiesser
Author photo by Amanda Clark
Edited by Danielle Sosin
Book design by Chelsea Bobula

Printed and distributed by Ingram
First edition 2022.

10 9 8 7 6 5 4

www.chefjillianforte.com

Duluth, MN

Printed in USA

Dedicated to Aurora.
If you dream it,
you can do it.

preface

On my first visit to At Sara's Table Chester Creek Cafe (ASTCCC), I was a 24-year-old college grad with a Costa Rican tan. Heartbroken, I was living in my parent's attic with no car, a few hundred bucks to my name, and a baby on my hip. I needed a job, a house, and a plan. A pretty classic description of a line cook "between jobs."

It was a cool Duluth day when I walked under the Taran's Marketplace sign and through the Cafe's entryway splattered with posters and notices. The waiting area held a self-serve coffee station, a ratty green couch, and a charming quirkiness. It was, however, the kitchen that drew my eye—the bustle, the shining stainless steel coolers, the grill, flat top, and sauté station. I believe the kitchen is the heart of the home.

This holds true in a restaurant as well, but multiplied by 50, and hopped up on caffeine. That day I watched the kitchen staff at work, a familiar timed dance, the juggling of sauté pans, plating, garnishing, and setting hot plates in the window. To me, it's a beautifully choreographed dance.

I've always been drawn to food and cooking. As a child, I watched my Cuban abuelita preparing yellow rice and chicken for big family gatherings. I imitated her by mushing up honeysuckle berries in my frisbee and recording segments of "Jillian's Cooking Show." As a near-adult, I tried the real deal as a prep/bartender on the Gunflint Trail. When I moved out west, I applied for more kitchen work. I justified continuing this "get through college" job as a way to further study anthropology, this time through food.

Half a dozen restaurants later, I got hired at three-year-old ASTCCC. I immediately noticed the differences. The owners were women, a first for me, and both the front and back of the house staff were balanced in gender. The typical "bro" kitchen culture seemed minimal. There was a small garden planted out front, with plans for a larger one in the parking lot. The restaurant composted, bought from local farmers, and made all of its food from scratch. The menu offered world-influenced cuisine, with the staff encouraged to contribute to specials. In short, I'd found my dream restaurant!

As time passed, I progressed in my culinary career learning tricks of the trade alongside discoveries about myself. The culture there confirmed my insights about my connection to the earth and my community, nurturing my sense of purpose, and ever-burgeoning passion for food. I learned to listen to the nuances of a sizzling pan and actively listen to my coworkers' feelings and ideas. I learned that foods that grow well together often taste great together. Much like people in a nurturing environment, support each other's growth. I learned to cook proteins low and slow, releasing a smooth depth of flavor. While hot and fast heat tightens the proteins, lending a toughness, an apt metaphor for drama and flaring tempers. I discovered each lesson like an ingredient to use in a recipe for good living. Cooking at ASTCCC became my path to discovering how I wanted to be in this world, my practical guidebook to building a value system.

'Right livelihood,' is the Buddhist principle "... *that each person should follow an honest occupation which fully respects other people and the natural world. It means being responsible for the consequences of our actions, and taking only a fair share of the earth's resources."* *(rightlivlihood.org)* 'Right livelihood,' felt to me like the foundation of the Cafe. The culture that Barb and Carla aimed to create was based on respect for their employees, connection to the greater community, and a demonstrated compassionate use of the earth. They were building a restaurant conscious of the consumption of resources like electricity and water, conscious of waste as witnessed in its composting practices. Their food network focused on sourcing local, nutrient-rich, and artfully crafted foods. At the restaurant, I felt I was part of a larger web of thought and action, of 'right livelihood' that resulted in offering the community a welcoming place to gather and eat wholesome meals.

By 2009, I was running the kitchen with the support of Barb and Carla. The Ladies gave me space to envision, and then build, a work environment that was positive, uplifting, and fun (OK, not all the time!) They encouraged me to find my voice and lead, and also delegate when needed. They helped me grow comfortable as a spokesperson in interviews and in front of TV cameras. They provided me with concrete learning opportunities like sending me to the Culinary Institute of America to deepen my knowledge of food and wine pairings, and they green-lighted my dream of offering offsite table-to-farm dinners. I felt free and empowered to play and experiment.

Now, 17 years after I began, and thousands of miles from Duluth, I sit at one of many desks, in as many towns across Mexico, to pen this cookbook. From this distance, I look back at all that transpired. Some memories have diminished, but others rise like stacks of bright-white plates under heat lamps. So many skills and lessons learned, both in and out of the kitchen. In truth, I grew up under the Cafe's roof.

The babe on my hip that first day as I stood outside ASTCCC is now a young woman, off on adventures of her own. Barb and Carla respected my role as a mother at the Cafe. Despite the demands of running a kitchen, my daughter came first. Aurora, too, grew up within those walls. She waited there for the school bus each day, spent afternoons working on homework in a booth, and helped Diane Bailey, the baker for 19 years, when she was curious about baking cookies. As a teenager, she even worked in the back of the house. The restaurant's culture, and its cast of characters, influenced both of us to become the women we are today.

The year 2022 celebrates At Sara's Table Chester Creek Cafe's 20th anniversary. This book is a tribute, a culinary memoir, to ASTCCC and to Barb Neubert and Carla Blumberg, the two bold women whose values wove the colorful fabric that is the culture of the restaurant. It is a history honoring my co-workers over the years, local purveyors, farmers, and customers. Their combined passions, quirks, talents, and energy created a place that many consider a community institution. To me, the Cafe feels like home.

Like others before me, I want to share my professional home kitchen with the home cook. My hope, my heart's genuine desire, is to spread the joy I find in cooking. That joy and satisfaction start with mindset. I ran the ASTCCC kitchen with these overarching ideas. Perhaps they can be helpful to you. Be *thoughtful* as you choose your ingredients. Look for quality items from your garden, the farmers' market, grocery store or butcher. Indulge in the *pleasure* of silky feeling flour, velvety peach skins or crispy bacon. Be *mindful* when slicing through fresh fruits and vegetables, smelling the sweetness, and crunching the juicy flesh. Take *pride* in the skill of flipping an over-easy egg, spatchcocking a chicken, and even simply emulsifying a vinaigrette by hand. Find *finesse* in finishing multiple elements for a meal at the same time. See the *art* in composing a plated meal with peaks of toast points and dollops of sauce. Appreciate the absolute crowning moment of sitting down with friends and family and eating within *community.* My favorite part of eating is sharing it with my loved ones. I encourage you to invite friends over and cook them your favorite dish from At Sara's Table Chester Creek Cafe!

I hope this book creates the same joy in your life that preparing these dishes over the years has in mine.

Chef Jillian

The secret ingredient is always love

contents

introduction

Tucked away in a slice of Duluth, Minnesota's Chester Bowl neighborhood, At Sara's Table Chester Creek Cafe (ASTCCC) has grown from a small restaurant and coffee shop into a community powerhouse and a popular destination for tourists and locals alike. Customers pack the dining room daily to enjoy a menu of new and exciting dishes and well-loved comfort foods. The restaurant's commitment to locally sourced ingredients, environmentally friendly practices, and an inclusive atmosphere set an inviting table. For 20 years, the Cafe has not only survived but thrived, a feat in the service industry and a testament to the owners' Barb Neubert and Carla Blumberg's vision. This cookbook tells the Cafe's herstory and features the voices of a host of dynamic characters employed at the Cafe over the years. They are the authors of recipes, contributors to the Professional Tips, tellers of tales and illustrators. Some have written heartfelt notes about working at the restaurant, and what 'the Ladies' (Barb and Carla) meant to them.

These pages offer a bounty of incredible recipes! Much like the Cafe menu, you'll find them organized into seven sections—Breakfast, Lunch, Dinner, Small Plates, Salads, Soups, and Baked Desserts. Ninety-plus recipes in all. As the volume cooked in restaurants far exceeds one's needs at home, each has been reduced to an appropriate size before testing. There are classics no longer on the menu but still asked for, like the Hummus and Tzatziki from the Mediterranean Plate. And there are signature "lifers" like the Hippie Farm Breakfast and the ever-popular Thai Curry. If you're new to the restaurant, you've got some exploring to do and regulars will take pleasure in finding their favorite gems.

The recipes in each section are presented with everything needed to prepare the dishes successfully and to your dietary needs. Each contains the overall time to prepare, serving size, needed equipment, and allergen information. In order to showcase our team of chefs past and present, the creator of each recipe is listed below the title. Also noted are hard-to-find ingredients, suggested substitutions, and alternative processes and equipment. Sprinkled throughout the book's pages are references to the 'Tips, Tricks, & Advice' section aimed to bolster your cooking success. For those with dietary and allergy concerns, each recipe is cited as gluten-free, vegetarian, vegan, and dairy-free, with any substitutions or omissions to meet those requirements. The book also includes an allergy index to make it easy to find dishes that match specific diets.

Note that the Dinner and Salad sections differ in format from the others (and most cookbooks!) It's written to allow the cooking of a single component or to construct the entire meal as served at the Cafe. Timing Notes 🔔 have been included to help you work through the steps of multiple/simultaneous recipes efficiently.

When you're ready to cook, start by setting up a well-lit, clean workspace. Consider putting on your favorite playlist or whatever brings you joy. Read through the recipe from start to finish, note the various Pro Tips, and then gather all the tools and ingredients a.k.a. your Mise en Place. Taste each ingredient as you prepare it. And remember, recipes are a guide to flavor profiles and amount ratios. They are inspirational, not the law. (With exceptions for baking!) Follow your intuition. Write any changes on the pages. Play with your food. Laugh at the mistakes. Most importantly, give thanks and have fun!

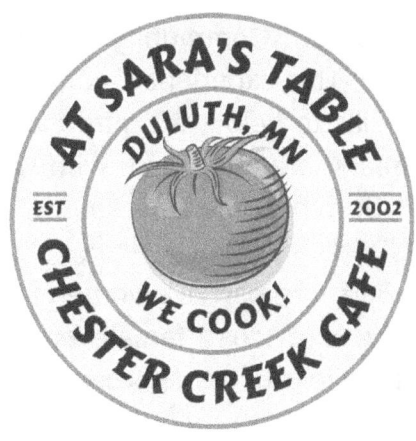

her-story

BARB'S STORY

Barbara Ann Neubert grew up on the shores of Lake Superior. In her early years, she enjoyed farm-fresh food grown and prepared on her grandparents' homesteads. These farm experiences formed many of her beliefs about food and health. Her German maternal grandmother worked on the family farm and cooked at home, while her paternal grandmother cooked professionally in local diners, inspiring Barb's dream of owning her own restaurant. These grandmothers taught Barb the healing qualities of whole foods and to appreciate a quality cup of coffee shared with family and friends.

After graduating from Duluth East High School, Barb enrolled at the University of MN, Duluth. Two years into her studies, she married and soon gave birth to her only child, Shelly. Barb dropped out of college to focus on her daughter. After becoming a single parent, she took night classes for her generals. At 32, Barb graduated with a degree in Urban Planning (a degree which she credits in choosing the At Sara's Table Chester Creek Cafe location). Her first "real job" was with the United Way as the bookkeeper for Duluth Community Health Center, a free clinic primarily serving women. This experience, combined with her planning degree, gave her the skills to help start a free family planning clinic in Superior, Wisconsin. Years later, her work with women inspired her to return to school. At 48, Barb became a nurse.

Throughout the 1970s, Barb was part of a women's consciousness-raising group that met weekly to discuss female empowerment. Feminism became her guiding principle or, as she describes it, her "north star."

This ritual of gathering with women to drink coffee and discuss life inspired Barb to write the novel, *At Sara's Table*. A name she would reuse throughout her life.

While at an outdoor music festival in the early 1990s, Barb and her girlfriend Mary Ann Rich watched people line up at a truck that served coffee. On the cusp of a trend that would define 90s American culture, the couple converted an old trailer into a traveling espresso shop which quickly built a reputation at local events and fairs. Becoming business owners allowed the couple to manage their health limitations while giving them the power to control their own lives.

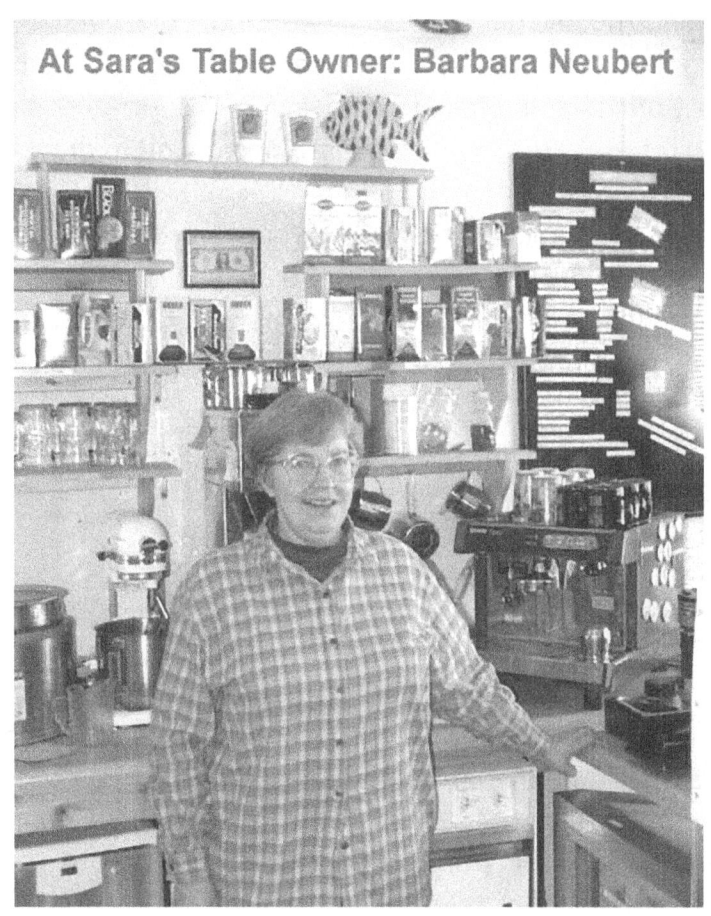
At Sara's Table Owner: Barbara Neubert

In 1994, the business went brick and mortar, and At Sara's Table got its start as a very small, poorly financed women's bookstore and coffeehouse. Barb says, "We borrowed money from my parents and sold our motorcycles and camping trailer to remodel an ugly, too small, but appropriately placed storefront overlooking Lake Superior on Superior Street." Though they hired out the technical work on the storefront, Barb proudly did all the carpentry. When she called a book contact and announced she had $300 to purchase a list of popular lesbian and feminist books, the woman laughed and told her the amount wasn't enough to start a bookstore and hung up! Opening the store proved expensive and difficult. Still,

ASTCCC was a humble way to further the Feminist movement, but for local teenager Jackie Fontaine (prep cook ASTCCC), the simple awareness of At Sara's Table's existence helped her feel connected to a queer community during a confusing period in her life.

they realized the bookstore/coffee shop dream, hosting after-hours meetings of women's groups and becoming a place that aspiring writers liked to frequent as they crafted their sentences. "The shop was rewarding," Barb recalled, "but it wasn't paying the bills." When the couple started serving soup and sandwiches, their earnings began to grow.

The small shop expanded into the space next door. One day, Carla Blumberg showed up as a volunteer to help with construction. She surveyed the situation, then picked up a hammer and quickly built the closets. The speed and efficiency of Carla's work impressed Barb, who told her, "If I ever have to be homeless, I would choose to be homeless with you." Her comment intrigued Carla. It was the spark that would one day lead to a wedding in their very own Chester Gardens.

CARLA'S STORY

Carla Ann Blumberg was born in Massachusetts, though her family soon relocated to Texas. "It was a terrible and memorable grief," Carla said, "for me to give up my snowsuit to move to a hot place." Though her German heritage was her predominant culinary influence, living so close to the southern border, she learned to prefer Mexican food. "German food was just *not cool*, growing up," she said.

Carla graduated from a segregated high school in 1964, the year Congress passed the Civil Rights Act. Her high school sweetheart was handsome, popular, and the class president, though they were both in the closet to all but close friends. Later, when Carla came out at home, her parents banned her from the house for 2 years.

After high school, Carla worked at the local newspaper and seriously considered studying journalism. She then worked for a while as a telephone operator for Southwestern Bell. It was an exciting world filled entirely with women, but she became bored when she realized women couldn't move up the ladder. She then earned an English degree from Texas Lutheran College and attended two years of summer school at San Francisco State University, where she studied theater lighting and design. In the late 60s, she moved from Berkeley to New York City to work for the Magic Theatre Company. "I was sleeping on a couch in the theater with a band of speed freaks living above me. It was overwhelming." Sick, and unable to find a doctor, she returned to Texas and resolved to spend time in nature.

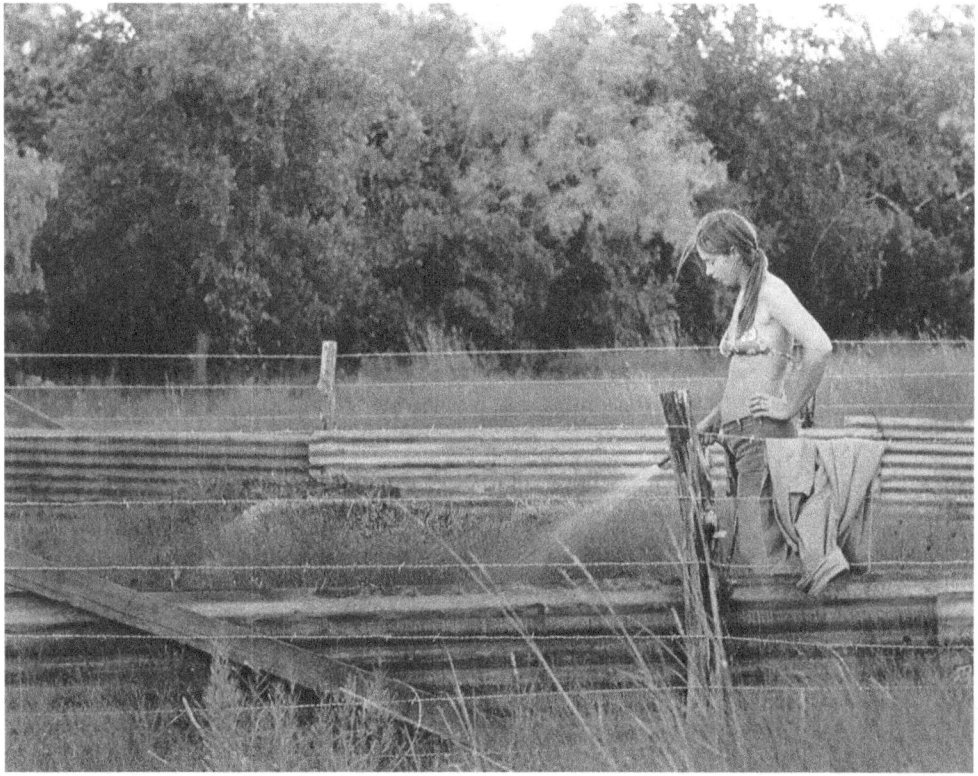

In the thick of the "Back to the Land" movement, Carla used a bit of money from her granddad to buy a dusty pasture. "In those days, everyone was about changing the world. We didn't get very far." She built a little kitchen shack, then a 1 bedroom cabin with hand tools and repurposed lumber. With no gardening experience nor ambition to be a farmer, she focused on improving the health of the soil. "I spent the entire time shoveling truckloads of animal manure and cotton trash," she said. After 5 years,

DANGEROUS DARCEE DOUGLAS

Carla's good friend Darcee helped as a handyperson at both Carla's restaurant and later at ASTCCC. It turns out that this soft-spoken woman was pretty famous in the Austin area. Carla recalled watching TV when someone on World of Wrestling lifted a man and threw him out of the ring. Looking closely, she realized it was Darcee! Years later, Max Moen, a beloved dishwasher at the Cafe who had lived in Austin, rounded the corner to find a towering woman tinkering with a broken shelf and exclaimed "Are you Dangerous Darcee Douglas?!"

Carla decided to learn the science behind the work and enrolled at the University of Texas, Austin, where she earned a degree in Molecular Biology.

In 1984, Carla bought a cheap old wreck of a farmstead in Austin and opened 'Carla's', her first restaurant. She grew vegetables on the acre out back and hired French-trained chefs, who taught her about line cooking and creating small-batch, high-end entrées. The clientele was primarily Austin lesbians and business folk. People would ask her, "Is it true that men can't come in here?" Though everyone was welcome, one guy threatened, "I'm going to come over there with my 38 and teach you all a lesson." "Typical Texas," Carla recalled. The business crashed with the stock market in 1987. Though the restaurant didn't last long as Carla's, it continued as a woman-run restaurant and a pioneer in recycling and composting for nearly two decades.

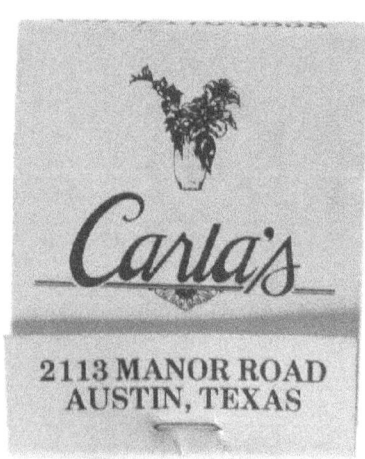

In the late 90s, while planning a road trip with her girlfriend, Carla looked at a map of the country. She saw Lake Superior's Isle Royale and thought it looked like an inviting destination. The couple made it as far as Two Harbors. While out getting firewood in the crisp night air, Carla looked up at the stars and knew she found the place she wanted to be. It was time to buy a new snowsuit.

When Sonja (server) thinks about her years as a server, she says it's easy to think she is just a server but really "Making people happy, that's what I do for a job. I make people happy, feel welcome, and comfortable."

Car accidents on the corner of the 19th and 8th are very common in the winter. "Coffee bar had this amazing view of cars sliding through the stop sign coming down 19th. Customers would grab a cup of coffee, sit in the comfy chairs and watch all the accidents." Faith Woodruff. There is a cringe-worthy YouTube compilation of cars sliding through this very intersection called "Icy Intersection". It also has a historic view of the architectural building before it was Chester Gardens.

the story of at sara's table chester creek cafe

THE BUILDING

Excited to set down roots in Duluth, Carla built a Norwegian-themed hotel and restaurant on the west end of Park Point, just over the Aerial Lift Bridge. Barb and Carla's budding romance was taking off, and they soon moved At Sara's Table from Superior Street into the dragon peaked building that Carla had constructed. "I imagined development just going all the way down that strip," Carla said, but her dream of expanding hit roadblocks, and the couple began looking for a new location.

Barb discovered that the historic Taran's Market Place, at 1902 East 8th Street, was for sale. Near two colleges, and at a trafficked intersection, Barb knew the location would be perfect. She was right. However, the structure had to be taken down to the foundation. Instead of calling in a wrecking ball, Barb and Carla salvaged as much of the building material as possible.

Carla and Emily Little, an architect friend from Austin, designed the new restaurant. Together, they created a dining room with beautiful flow boasting tall windows that faced Lake Superior. The high ceiling beams, booths, benches, and the 10' tall bookshelves in the room called 'the library,' a tribute to At Sara's Table bookstore, were crafted from the wood salvaged from Taran's Market Place and the Park Point property.

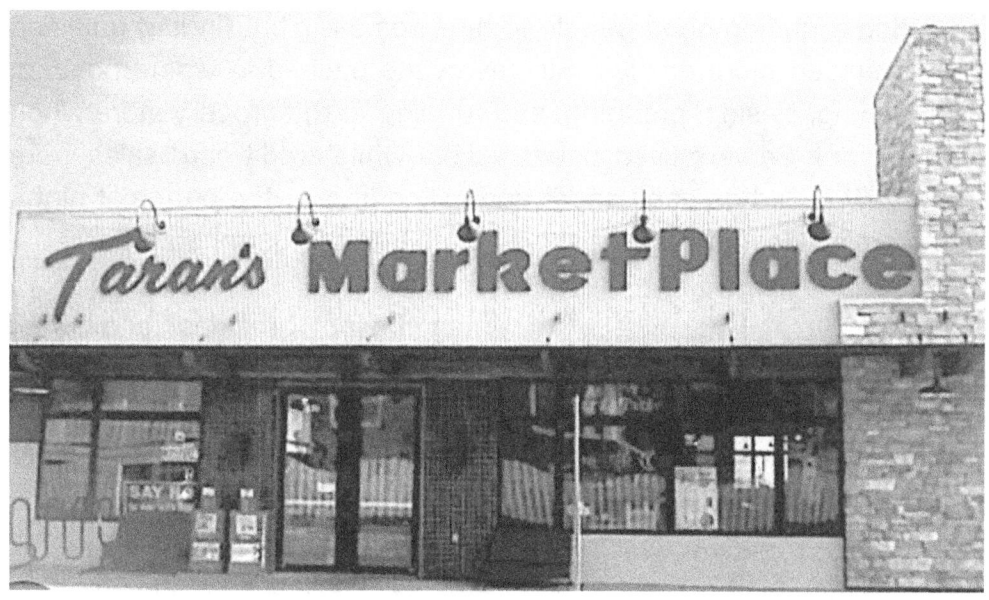

WHAT'S IN A NAME, ANYWAY?!

Barb and Carla (the Ladies) kept the Taran's Market Place sign, a familiar landmark for the community, with a plan that the building would be multi-use and hold various businesses. The idea was short-lived. The Market Place sign led to much confusion from passers-by who came looking for a grocery store only to find a restaurant. For Barb, the name At Sara's Table was a tribute to her novel, the coffee truck, and her bookstore/coffee house. She felt it important to keep a recognizable and reputable name in order to bring along her clientele. Together, the two chose the name Chester Creek Cafe, signaling the restaurant's location. Thus, the business ended up with three names when it opened on October 15th, 2002.

An elderly man lived up the street and had grown up shopping at Taran's Market Place. In the restaurant's early years, he came by regularly to buy milk and eggs. Carla insisted the staff sell him whatever he wanted.

The Ladies, basing their business expectations on their solo forays of the past, crafted an initial menu of soups, salads, bakery items, and coffee drinks. Nothing prepared them for the immediate and immense popularity of the Cafe. Carla prepped, cooked, and did the ordering, hiring, and scheduling, while Barb managed all the front-of-the-house operations. Finding good people to hire was easy, but finding qualified people proved more difficult. Still, everyone pitched in where needed: dishwashing, closing, prepping, and running to the grocery store when food ran out. Servers used paper tickets while credit card sales were "rung up" on carbon copy paper and called in over the phone at night. "We were just learning the hard way, all the way through," said Barb.

"It was really stressful for the Ladies in the early years, but they tried really hard to take care of the employees. They rented houses to us, found healthcare for us, not to mention paid us well."
- Kelly Rubel (FOH manager)

When the hot breakfast and lunch menu began, The Hippie Farm Breakfast 37, inspired by Carla's farm days debuted. It is still a popular menu item today. In time, Carla envisioned adding a dinner service of haûté cuisine similar to the offerings at her restaurant in Austin. She hired classically trained Bruce Wallis (head chef), who set the stage for things to come with his unique flavor combinations. Peter Ravinski (operations manager) remembers how the menu changed daily. "We'd get this bag of veggies from the Food Farm and make something. If it lasted three days, great. If not, we'd have to come up with something different." Night chef Colleen Betts recalled the process being "fun and super creative." For a period Carla created regional menus such as 'The Rhine River,' 'Andalusia,' and 'The Pacific Northwest.' "I don't know if we expanded our dinner population by doing all those crazy things," Barb said, "but... I kind of miss those days."

The Cafe's increasing popularity and standing in the community created a need for more physical space. Originally, prep cooking, baking, line cooking, and dishwashing all occurred within the view of customers. It was a tight squeeze. The first order of expansion became an official prep room, allowing space to prepare higher volumes of food. The prep team quickly dubbed the new room 'Serenity Central,' as it allowed the staff some behind-the-scenes breathing room. Next, they doubled the original patio to its current size. The additional tables were a blessing, though Duluth's notoriously changeable weather sent servers chasing airborne menus, guest checks, and even oversized deck umbrellas down the street. A major change came about when Carla redesigned the basement to house both the bakery and a private room to be used for book clubs, parties, and meetings. Next, the kitchen was bumped outward into the newly expanded parking lot. Rita Bergstedt (gardener) built and planted the first ASTCCC garden near the corner of the lot where Barb housed the new genuine Texas smoker she'd bought. Hello, smoked salmon!

I continue to enjoy my relationship both on a personal level and business level with the Chester Creek Cafe—The two seem to have melded. We share words or sit down together and have wonderful meals. I've been given advice on my own personal life as my transitions continue, shared stories amidst laughter and joy, always mindful of the wonderful food, and left full in the richest of ways.
- Dave Rogotzke (salmon supplier & friend)

"We appreciate the reliability of the working relationship (with ASTCCC) that has evolved over the years."
- John Fisher-Merrit (Food Farm)

Carla believes that buying locally and sustainably procures the freshest food while lowering the carbon footprint and keeps money in the community. Paired with Barb's business philosophy based on creating dependable relationships they have built an enduring locally supplied network for ASTCCC. Farm friendships include:

Dave Rogotzke's Simple Gifts, Food Farm, Birch Point Gardens, Yker Acres, Bay Produce, Amish Farmers, Ashland Baking Company, Duluth's Best Bread, 3rd Street Bakery, Johnson's Bakery, Jeremy Frisee, 1,000 Hills, Larry Schultz Organic Eggs, Kadejan Farms. For beverages, the Ladies chose B&W Coffee Roasters, Anahata Herbals, Bent Paddle, Castle Danger and Earth Rider Breweries, Carlos Creek Winery, Vikre Distillery, Panther Distillery, Prairie Vodka, Du Nord Social Spirits, Crooked Waters Spirits, and Tattersall Distillery. The Cafe also prides itself on buying from local foragers and neighbors who bring their offerings to the kitchen doors!

DID YOU KNOW?

Did you know? There are no lines painted in the parking lot because it is four inches short of having two legal-sized rows down the center. Committing that much space would have required the beautiful maple tree by the garden to be cut down.

BARB'S BABY, THE BAR

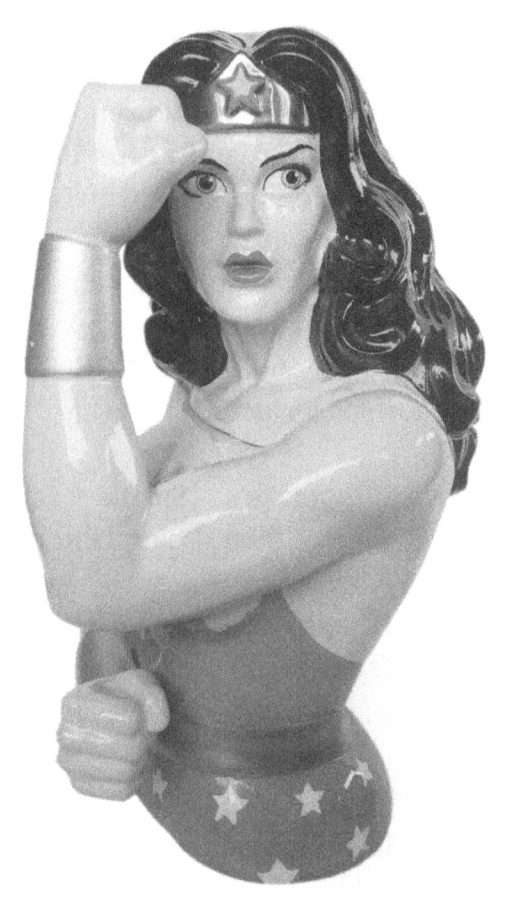

When Barb and Carla's only tenant, a real estate company, moved out of the building, Barb didn't hesitate - the space was perfect for a bar! With the help of Amy Nakamura (finish carpenter) and the famous Darcee Douglas (handy person), the team designed and built the intimate dark-hued bar and booths. Barb found a mirrored bar back, purchased the Hamm's beer sign secondhand, and chose the feminist-leaning art, including the large painting by Steph Richards (server) that hangs prominently above the bar.

The bar opened in 2009, with a license to serve beer and wine. In time, Sarah Maxim (server/wine rep) and Carey Kasapidis (FOH manager) created a memorable wine list. They aimed to serve sustainable wines from producers operating with organic and/or biodynamic farming and winemaking

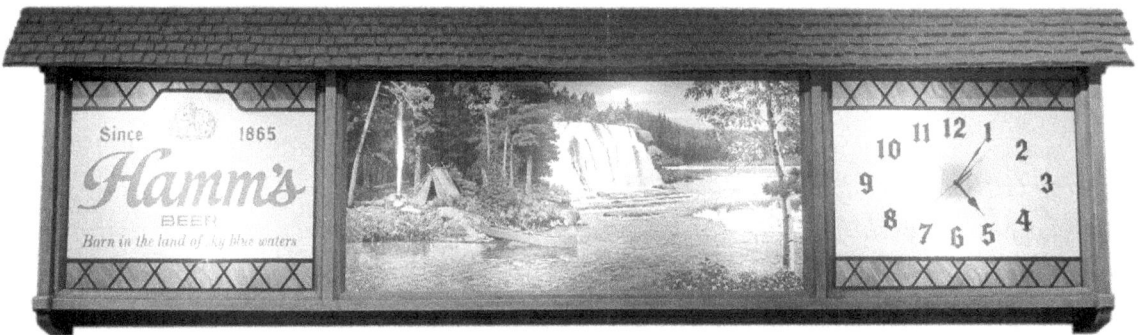

DID YOU KNOW?

The most coveted item by cafe customers is the Hamm's beer sign, closely followed by the Wonder Woman cookie jar.

practices. They also sought out women-owned and operated companies and winemakers. Eventually, the restaurant obtained a full liquor license, opening the door to more complex drinks, and arguably wilder events!

Barb's vision created a much-loved space used for quiet evenings out, staff meetings, and raucous parties. It's common to find Barb and/or Carla eating dinner in the corner booth, or Sharla Gardner (office), a long-time friend and part-time employee, having a meal at the bar. The crew served Spam sushi in the bar at Barack Obama's celebratory inauguration party, and years later, took turns wandering in, teary-eyed, to watch Hillary Clinton's concession speech. The bar has hosted Saturday morning music during Duluth's yearly Homegrown Music Festival, serving hangover drinks to the festival-goers on their way to the notorious kickball game in Chester Bowl. There was also the weekly get-together Service Industry Night, or SIN as it's known, that caters to restaurant workers—the only night of the week employees could drink in the bar. As always, ASTCCC's bar hosts a steady stream of political meetings and events.

DID YOU KNOW?
Barb and Carla have donated to nearly 300 different local organizations, many of them yearly.

POLITICS AND BUSINESS? YES, WE CAN!
Though most business owners keep their personal beliefs out of their storefronts, Barb and Carla want the world to hear their message. Left-leaning signs are consistently present in the Cafe windows. 'Black Lives Matter.' 'We Believe in Science.' 'Happy Pride.' 'Blessed Ramadan.' The most controversial sign has been 'Get Out of Iraq' produced by faculty members of UMD. Though occasionally there has been backlash, Barb and Carla have stood their ground. "I felt we wouldn't lose any of our valued customers," Barb said, knowing the political bent of most of her diners. Peter Ravinski (operations manager) seconded this sentiment. "The people who gravitate here tend to believe in the restaurant's mission statement. I work here because the Cafe has a belief system that supports social and environmental justice."

Democracy must be something more than two wolves and a sheep voting on what to have for dinner.

James Bovard

MISSION STATEMENT

At Sara's Table Chester Creek Cafe is a farm-to-table restaurant. We pay attention to where and who our food comes from and how it is handled. We are interested in the health and welfare of individual animals and in the environment as a whole. Our cooking style is focused on quality rather than output. We pay our employees a living wage and treat them with respect. We are community-oriented and regard our customers as partners in the creation of a comfortable and supportive environment attentive to the culinary and social needs of those we serve.

Barb and Carla's political beliefs have also shaped the internal policies of the restaurant. Their feminism is born of a deep understanding of issues facing women, LGBTQ, and gender expansive folx. The Cafe's goal is to be an inclusive culture and safe environment for all. Managers, frequently women, encourage preferred pronoun usage and appearance. They inform new employees about standards and expectations of the work culture, including the Cafe's proactive sexual harassment policy designed to stop harassment before it gets out of line. Of course, life at the Cafe is not perfect. It's still a restaurant with real people, messy complicated issues, and plenty of drama, but the intent and awareness to be respectful and act in kindness is part of the everyday fabric.

The phrase "topic change" when spoken by any employee immediately stops conversation, no questions asked. This empowers individuals to express discomfort without having to explain their reasoning at the moment.

St. Louis River Alliance

Randy Marshall
Environmental Stewardship Award

Presented to

*At Sara's Table
Chester Creek Cafe*

For exemplary efforts to protect the St. Louis River and Lake Superior through conscientious environmental business practices

Diane R. Nelson
SLRA Chair

Jack Ezell
Chair, Stewardship Committee

ST. LOUIS RIVER
ALLIANCE

April 2011

LOVELY LUSH ORGANIC GARDENS

In 2014, Carla and Emily Little designed a multi-use building and garden on 19th Ave, diagonal from the Cafe. The corner once held a Standard gas station, followed by an architectural firm. By the time Carla tore down the building, the city considered the land a polluted "brown site." In order to repair the damage, she had the contaminated soil removed and brought in clean fill. The city awarded her for Brown Field Remediation.

In a lovely effort to remediate and cycle nutrients through the soil, Carla created a garden. Rita Bergstedt (gardener), and Darcee Douglass (handy person), built the three-tiered Chester Garden. The space is large enough to keep two gardeners busy, but the amount of food it produces barely makes a dent in the needs of the busy restaurant. As a result, Rita chose to plant more expensive and difficult-to-source vegetables. "I felt that there were items that would thrive in this environment, and yet be unusual and a welcome addition to the Cafe's offerings," she said. Chester Garden reliably produces an array of blueberries and unique vegetable varieties that the chefs love to showcase in summer garden specials.

Chester Garden and the Cafe's parking lot garden add beauty while repairing two tiny corners of the city. They are not moneymakers, and their impact on local environmental health is minuscule, but like most of the restaurant's practices, the gardens demonstrate that the personal is political. Leading by example, Barb and Carla teach that all of our decisions are of consequence. The restaurant has composted food scraps from day one, eventually becoming a compost collection site for the neighborhood, and offering free compostable bags available at the coffee bar. The toilets are low flush, and the lights are on sensors to reduce electricity usage. Given global deforestation, even the restroom toilet paper is a sustainably harvested product. These small quiet choices, unseen by most, exemplify the guiding principles of ASTCCC.

NEVERTHELESS, SHE PERSISTED!

In 2018, Carla designed a remodel that would boost the restaurant's efficiency and solve multiple problems: more restrooms, increased cooler and freezer space, new equipment, an upgraded dishwashing area, as well as plans to build a third-floor conference room that would showcase a fabulous lake view. However, the remodel would require the restaurant to close its doors for a scheduled few weeks. The three-week closing turned into five. The Cafe excitedly reopened on Valentine's day 2020.

In March, the entire state went into pandemic lock down, and the doors of the restaurant closed again. By April, the restaurant was allowed to sell take out, but the inherent rules of the food game had changed. Fluctuating mandates and guidelines confused managers, staff, and customers. Food shortages and preventive employee time off proved to be a challenge. To survive, the restaurant needed to be flexible. The team stepped up, adjusted menus, wore masks, got vaccinated, and tried their best. Peter Ravinski (operations manager) and Amy Nakamura (finish carpenter) built an out-building for drive-through ordering and pickup and moved patio furniture to the parking lot to allow for more seating. Not one customer entered the building until mid-June 2020.

The primary concern throughout the pandemic was to keep everyone safe. Carla and Barb followed the rules and were strict with the staff and customers requiring masks long before the statewide mandate. In the first year and a half, only two employees got sick. Covid-19 never spread through the Cafe. Gratitude was the most common response from our customers, though some displayed anger yelling at servers and hosts. Restaurants had become the venting place for society's frustration. Our front-facing employees shed a lot of tears. For an array of reasons, people were leaving the industry. The once steady, flexible restaurant workforce dwindled. It became a scramble to fill the schedule and to get ingredients in the door.

Throughout the incredibly emotional difficulties of the pandemic, Carla was a consistent force of optimism and encouragement. Carey Kasipidis (FOH manager) understood the severity of the pandemic and took every precaution. With thoughtful leadership and committed staff, a safe space was created for our customers. Nevertheless, the Cafe persisted!

20 years!

Carla's original goal with the restaurant was to be of service to her community by providing jobs and supporting farmers. Barb's goal was born of feminist ideals which led her to promote women's upward mobility. Their shared and overlapping values created the unique framework that is At Sara's Table Chester Creek Cafe.

When Barb thinks back over the past 20 years of owning and running the restaurant, she says, "It has given me purpose, been fun, and added color to my life. It's something to put in my obituary. We have made a lot of friends and have contributed to the community we live in." Carla, ever the practical Virgo, says "I am glad that I was finally able to learn how to cook here–after 40 years of trying. I've genuinely enjoyed (most) of the people I have worked with. This place is my chance to make a dent in the world, this little corner." Carla and Barb's "dent in the world" is a beautiful legacy of supporting local farmers and community, creating opportunities, jobs, nurturing women leaders, and—oh yeah—serving up delicious food!

Happy 20th Birthday to At Sara's Table Chester Creek Cafe! And Many More!

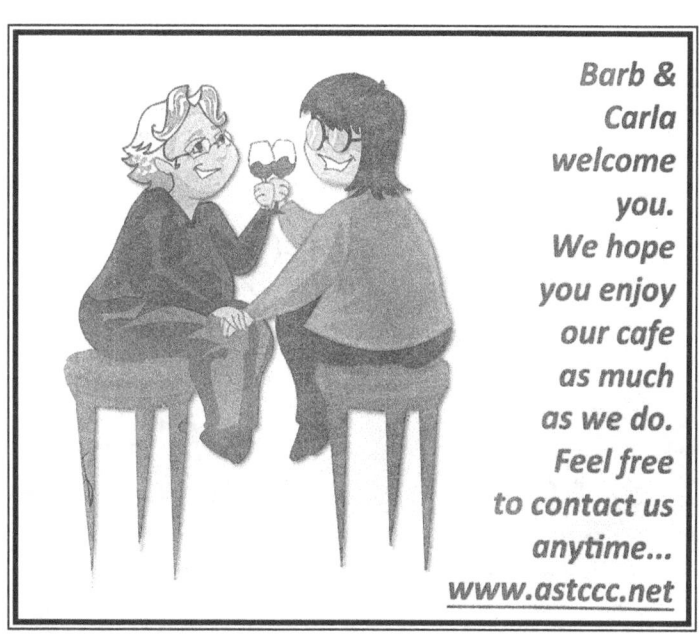

Barb & Carla welcome you. We hope you enjoy our cafe as much as we do. Feel free to contact us anytime... www.astccc.net

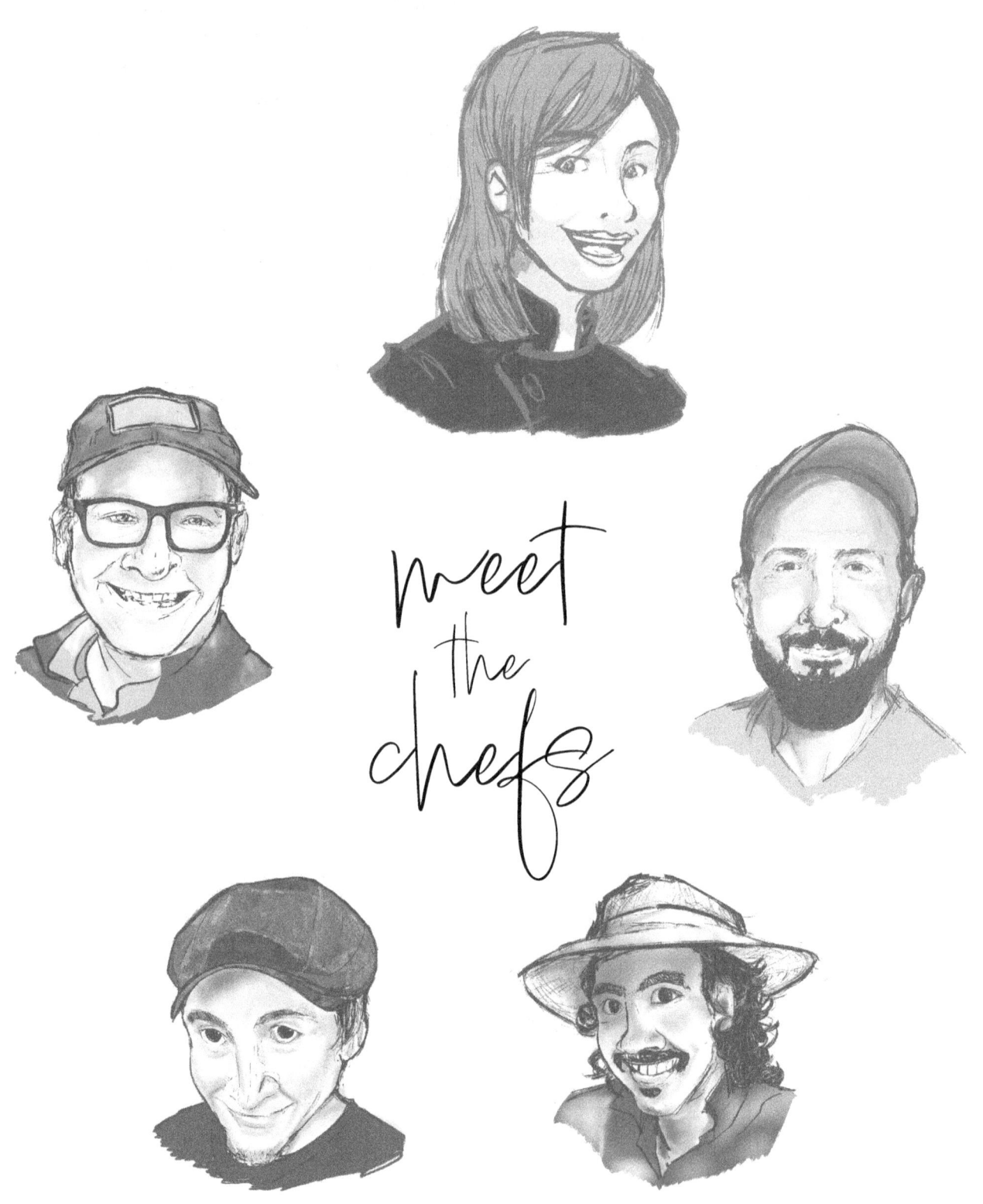

meet the chefs

ILLUSTRATED BY: CRISTINA PLASCENCIA *(HOST)*

tips, tricks, & advice

People who love to cook understand that in a kitchen there are always new techniques to master, ingredients to be discovered, and recipes to try. It's curiosity mixed with desire that makes for joyful learning and builds confidence. Throughout my 20 years of professional cooking, I have taught, yet never stopped being a student. I have learned a lot from my fellow line cooks, prep cooks, servers, and even dishwashers, which is why, after writing some tips and tricks, I reached out to them for their tidbits of wisdom. As usual, my coworkers did not disappoint! Though I'd planned to sprinkle tips and tricks throughout the book, the sheer abundance of my co-workers' sound advice demanded the creation of its own section. Some tips are practical, some encourage intuition and experimentation, while others speak to attitude. You can read through this collection or look up tips and tricks when referenced in a recipe. There is something here for everyone, even the professionals out there!

PAN TYPES

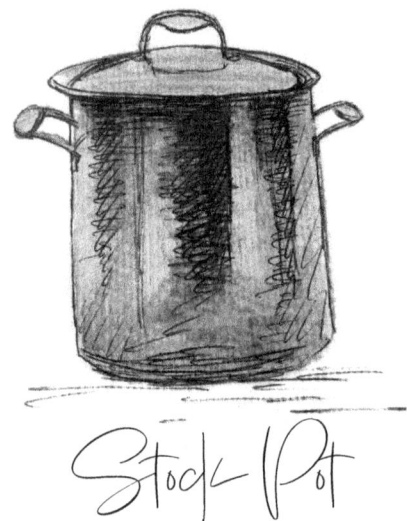

Stockpots preferably have a heavy-bottom so vegetables can be sautéed and then liquid added. Perfect for soups or stocks.

Stock Pot

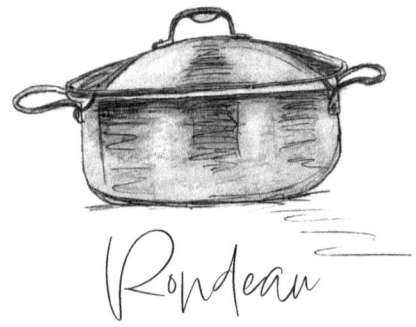

Rondeaus (aka brasier) have a "heavy-bottom" which disperses heat while cooking, making food less likely to scorch. The wider size of a rondeau also allows for searing meat without overcrowding. Having at least one heavy-bottom pot will create ease in successfully completing recipes that require sautéing, followed by the addition of liquids, like soup!

Rondeau

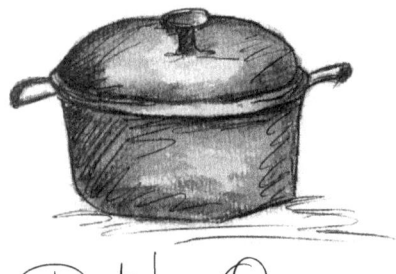

Dutch ovens are excellent for starting a recipe on the stove top then transferring to an oven. Dutch ovens hold heat evenly, and for a long time, making them perfect for a slow, low simmer, or bake.

Dutch Oven

   ILLUSTRATED BY: MELISSA WEISSER *(SERVER)*

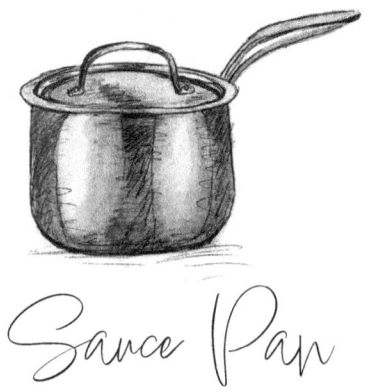

Sauce Pan

Sauce pans are versatile and excellent for cooking rice, sauces, poaching eggs, and reheating foods.

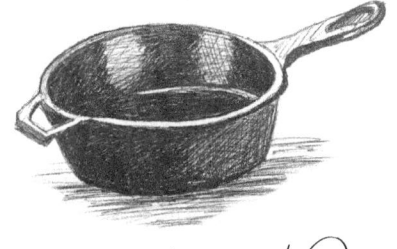

Cast Iron Pan

Deep cast-iron pans can be seasoned, creating a virtually nonstick pan, making them excellent for stovetop cooking. Their heavy thickness holds heat and provides a steady, even cooking base. The taller sided versions are great for stew.

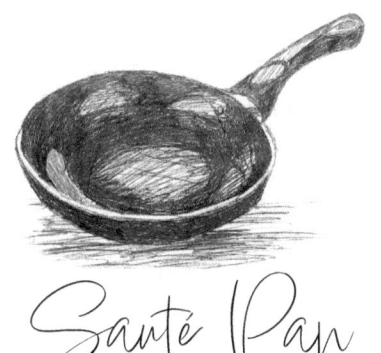

Sauté Pan

Sauté pans' curved lip lends itself to tossing and flipping food without the use of a spatula. It's important to remember that if your sauté pan is Teflon coated, use only rubber or silicone utensils. Plastic melts and metal will scrape the Teflon, reducing the pan's non-stick qualities and getting Teflon in your food.

BEFORE YOU START

Mistakes happen in the kitchen all the time. It's part of what helps us grow and learn about what works, and what we, as cooks, could do better next time. Don't ever let a mistake deter you. Giving up shouldn't be an option. You will grow and learn with each and every attempt. I'm a bit of a perfectionist. In the past, if I felt I didn't do something absolutely perfect to my liking, or others' liking, I used to just give up. That was, until one of my mentors gave me some much needed advice which was to keep going, keep trying, keep experimenting, and keep expanding my skill set. Cooking isn't always easy, but it can be extremely fun with the right mindset! - Hana Gaudreau (prep cook)

Snap a photo of recipes before you go shopping. It's easier than writing a list. But when you start cooking, have a pen handy and write in your cookbooks! Take notes of adjusted spice levels and cook times as you work through a recipe. Remember, a cookbook is a training manual, a workbook, and ultimately a guide. Feel free to change, add, or enhance any recipe, anywhere! - Jillian Forte (chef)

If you know someone who cooks for a living, you probably know someone who is more than mildly obsessed with towels. Most shifts start with the team standing in the laundry room folding and stacking the clean white squares to bring up the line. Douglas Adams' (author of Hitchhiker's Guide to the Galaxy) insistence that you "don't forget your towel" hits professional cooks on a spiritual level. Keep a dry one tucked into your apron strings or thrown over your shoulder, and I guarantee you'll find many uses for it in the kitchen. The less fancy and decorative your towels are, the more likely it is you'll use them, so stick to simple. - Ben Butter (line cook)

Always, always wash your hands very well before starting. Don't forget between your fingers and your wrists. Remember, it takes 30 seconds of scrubbing to get all the bacteria off. And wash EVERYTHING after touching proteins like chicken, beef, pork, and fish. This includes your cutting board and knife. Cross-contamination is easy to do and the consequences are a big bummer. - Jillian Forte (chef)

Feed the body, feed the mind. Put on music, or listen to a TED Talk. - Jackie Fontaine (prep cook)

Remember to always hone your knife before the start of each task. Believe it or not, you are more likely to cut yourself using a dull knife. - Casey Watsula (line cook)

If you have problems with your cutting board slipping, place a damp towel under it to keep it in place. Never use a glass cutting board. It will damage your knives and make for a frustrating experience. Keep a spray bottle with a mild bleach solution (¾ teaspoon bleach per 1-quart water) to disinfect your boards after use with raw meats. If you can, designate a specific cutting board to be used for meat, and one for ready-to-eat foods. - Channie McCall (line cook)

Don't have a diamond steel to straighten the edge of your knives? Use the bottom of a ceramic coffee cup instead. The grit in the clay or ceramic is usually just enough to flatten out the grooves on the knife edge. - Jillian Forte (chef)

"Mise en place (MEEZ ahn plahs). Everything in its place," my boss said to me in her doubly exotic English accent, being that I was a fresh implant to the coastal bend of south Texas. I was 18, a dishwasher, or "utility specialist" making the GIANT leap out of the dish pit, to become one of the staff whom I perceived as Rockstars... Mise en place is the practice of gathering all ingredients and utensils before you start preparing a dish. After handwashing, this was the most important kitchen practice ever taught to me. - Jackie Fontaine (prep cook)

Always keep dry pasta in the pantry. During my years working at an Italian restaurant, I was in charge of making sure everyone on the team was full and happy before dinner service started, but the expensive and important ingredients were off-limits. I had to get crafty and scrappy by using leftovers that were on the verge of being tossed. I learned from this daily challenge that most dishes can be reimagined and transformed with the help of pasta noodles! A staff favorite was pasta e fagioli, which translates to pasta and beans. Take your leftover beans (cannellini beans make it extra creamy), and heat them up with a couple of spoons of tomato sauce, some fresh chopped sage, garlic, and a dash of cayenne for spice. Toss in your noodles and enjoy. Bonus points. You didn't waste any food! - Chelsea Bobula (prep cook, graphic designer)

If you suddenly have unexpected dinner guests and not enough food, make extra rice or potatoes, throw together a quick garlic bread, or pop some bread rolls into the oven. Starches are a good way to fill a stomach. - Jillian Forte (chef)

PREPPING TIPS

Never scrape the blade side of your knife on a cutting board. This will only dull your edge and create more work sharpening. Use the back of the knife to pick things up from the cutting board, or just pick up the entire board and slide off the ingredients. - Bruce Wallis (head chef)

Place fresh thyme in a plastic tub and freeze for a minimum of 30 minutes before using. When ready to use, just shake the container and thyme leaves will come off of the stem. I hate de-stemming thyme. This really helps. It's a real... Thyme saver! - Rachel Anvary (prep cook)

Mince herbs by rocking the knife. Place your herbs in a tight pile in front of you, place your left hand on the tip of the knife, and press down. Move your right hand in a rocking motion slightly back and forth to mince the herbs. Chiffonade means to slice very thin. The best way to accomplish this with leafy herbs is to roll them into a manageable tube, (not super tight), and slice your way as thinly as possible down the tube. The first few cuts will probably be sloppy. By the middle, you will get the hang of it, and at the end, you'll risk your fingertips. Just let those pieces fly, or give them a little mince. - Jillian Forte (chef)

Use twice the amount of fresh herbs to replace dried, and subsequently half the amount of dried herbs to replace fresh. Why? The water has evaporated out of dried herbs, reducing their volume in half. When adding dried herbs to a recipe, place them in the palm of your hand and crush them into dust. This breaks the cell walls and frees the essential oils. If drying your own herbs, try to leave them in whole leaves to preserve the oils. - Jillian Forte (chef)

Cook with fresh ginger root. It can be cut into tablespoon-size chunks and stored in the freezer. - Danielle Sosin (prep cook)

Peeling garlic cloves the easy way. Lay the clove on your cutting board and put the flat side of your chef's knife on top. Use your palm to flatten the clove. Even just cracking the clove will make the skin come off lickety-split! - Jillian Forte (chef)

How much to prep? Vegetable sizes vary considerably and are tricky to measure in a measuring cup because of their cut shape. At home, I cut the veggies, mix them, then divide them into piles to gauge if it is an appropriate amount per person. This can be tricky because appetites vary. But if you know grandma eats like a bird and your construction worker uncle is coming to dinner, you can make their piles appropriately sized. Store any leftover veggies in the fridge, then add them to a pasta dish or stir-fry. Good Luck! - Jillian Forte (chef)

Tomato - What knife is best for cutting tomatoes? First, a little about knives. A chef's knife or a santoku (my favorite) has a straight sharp edge, thickening out for stability. The sharpness aids in smooth slicing and works well for chopping or mincing. A serrated knife is built like a saw and tears through fibers. It will never work for a chop because the scalloped edge only touches the cutting board intermittently. A serrated knife will leave a tomato's tender flesh with jagged edges. If the tomato will be cooked or mashed up, who cares?! But when showcasing the tomato, like on a Caprese, smooth edges reign. If your chef's knife won't easily slice through tomato skin, it's not sharp enough.

De-seeding a tomato - Slice the tomato in half through the center. Poke a finger into the seed pockets and scoop the seeds out over a compost bowl. This method keeps the shape of the tomato.

Potatoes - Ever notice that your vegetable peeler has a pointed tip? This is for digging out any eyes on a potato, or spots that go deeper than the peeler's blade. To prevent oxidation or browning of raw potatoes, cover them in water. Drain before use.

To peel or steam winter squash? Steaming is almost always the easiest way to deal with any variety of winter squash. Cut in half, de-seed, lay flesh side down on a sheet pan, add a splash of water and bake until soft. This gives you a great squash pulp excellent for purees. For nice bite-sized, chewy cubes, peel, dice, and bake.

REFERENCED TIPS

Juicing a lemon or lime - Before you slice the fruit, roll it on your cutting board, firmly pushing down with your palm to break the fruit's capillaries. Slice in half through the middle. To juice, use a manual juicer, or try my trick. Place a fine-mesh strainer over a measuring cup or bowl, then stick the tines of a fork into the flesh of the fruit and wiggle the fork handle up and down and around. This method yields a lot of juice and the strainer helps to keep those pesky seeds from slipping into the bowl.

Onions, julienned - Cut off the onion's root and stem. Slice the onion in half from the root to the tip. Peel. Place the onion flat-side down on the cutting board with the root side towards your stomach. Work from right to left (for righties) slicing the onion every ¼ -inch to create gently curving slivers.

Onion, finely diced - Cut off the onion's root and stem. Slice the onion in half from the root to the tip. Peel. Place the onion flat-side down on the cutting board with the root side pointed towards the right side of the cutting board. Holding the onion together, slice thin half-moons. Divide the slices into two halves. Place the center cut of the onion on the cutting board. Dice each quarter onion from one side to the other.

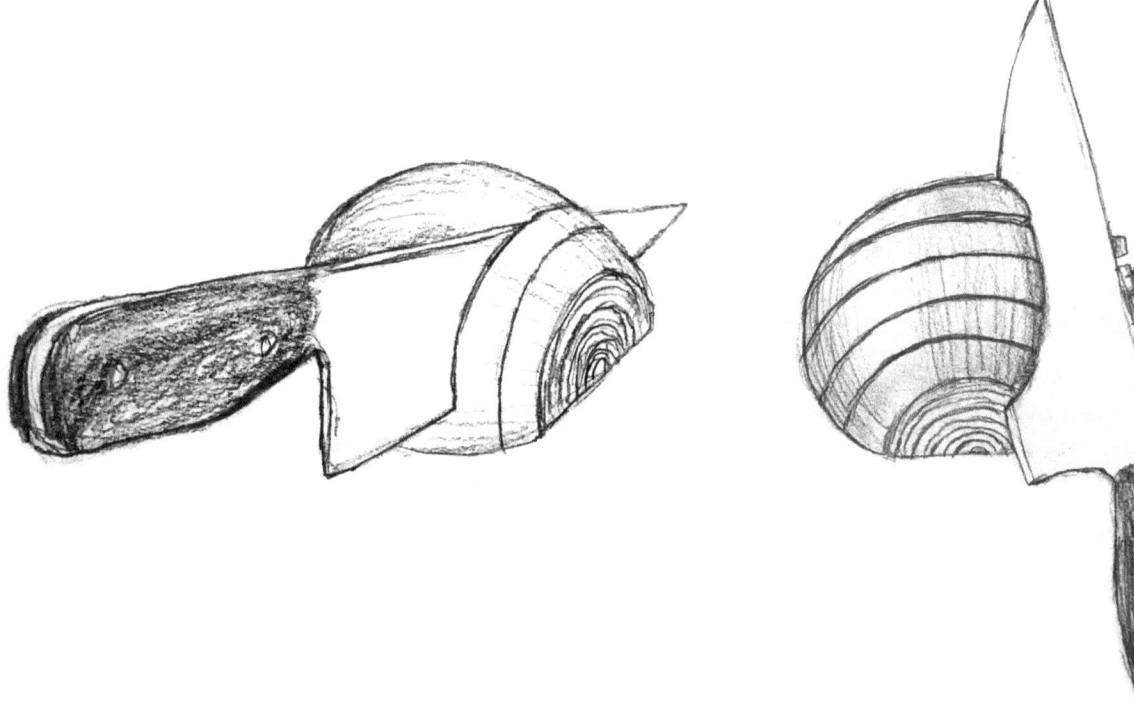

ILLUSTRATED BY: BENJAMIN ZABAN-BOYLAN (*LINE COOK*)

Peppers - Cutting peppers without disturbing the seed pod and getting seeds all over your cutting board is possible! Break or cut off the stem. Hold the pepper stem side down on the cutting board. Starting at the now top, slice off one side of the pepper, ending at the stem, approx. ¼ of the pepper. Remove the piece, now you can see inside. With each following slice, you can remove the white pith as well. Repeat, working your way around the pepper, while steering clear of the seed pod at the bottom. It should leave you with 4 pieces of pepper flesh with minimal white pith attached and a stem, seed pod, and pith in the other hand. Discard the seeds and pith, then slice or julienne the flesh.

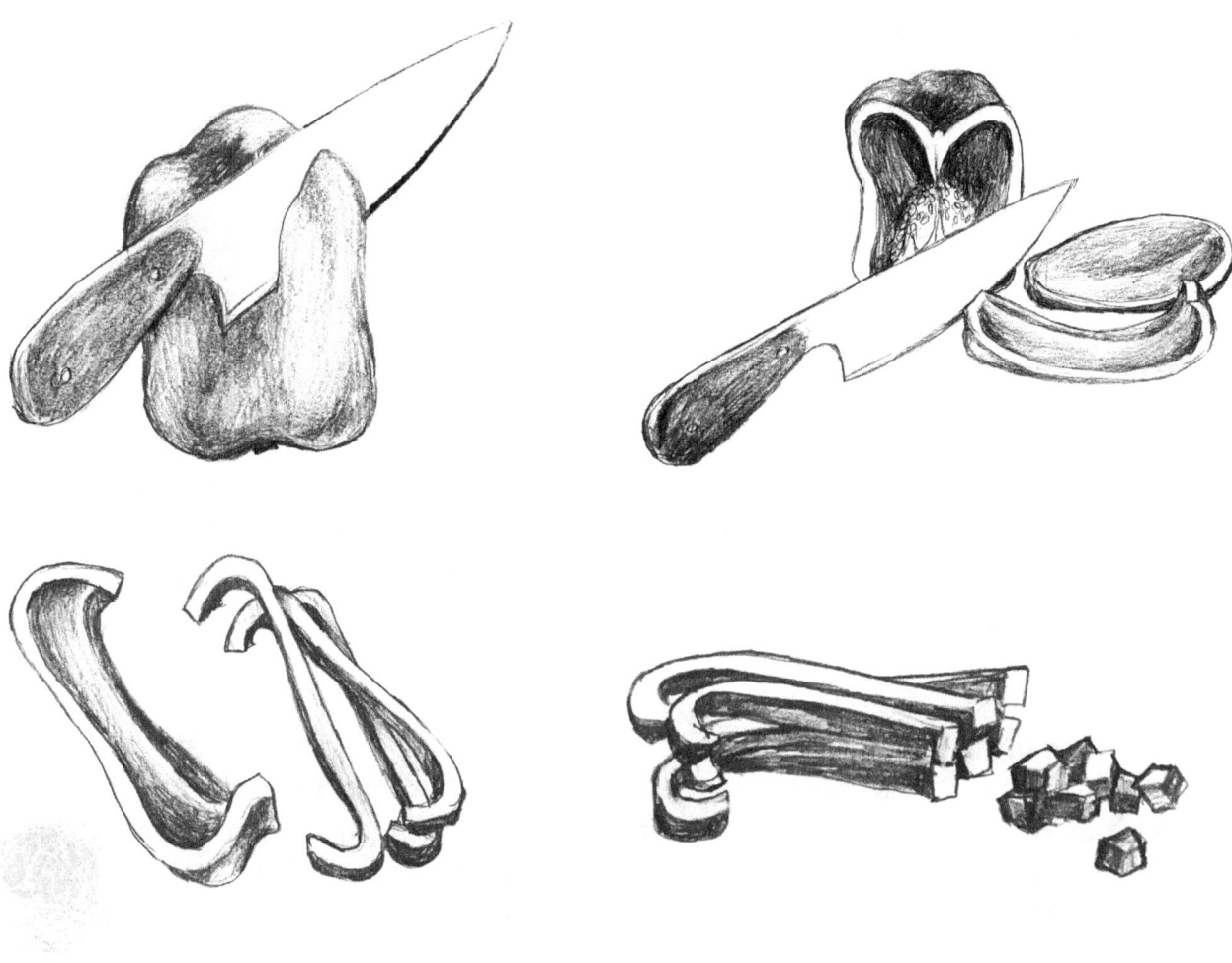

Kale - To de-stem all varieties of kale efficiently, hold on to the stem with one hand and run your thumb, pointer, and middle finger up the stem, ripping off the leaf as you go. This method works in one fell swoop.

Avocado - Slice the avocado from the stem to the bottom in a full circle. Grasp each side of the fruit and twist, pulling the fruit away from the pit. Hold the half with the pit in one hand and very carefully strike the heel of your knife into the center of the pit. It should stick to the pit. Now twist the knife, pull out the pit, and discard. (If this seems scary to you, take the side with the pit and gently push the skin beneath until the pit pops out.) Cupping the avocado in your hand, gently cut through the flesh, but not through the skin, to make slices. Now use a spoon to scoop out the slices.

Cherry Tomato halves - Place a plastic lid on top of a dozen or so cherry tomatoes. Gently hold the lid in place while you slide your knife parallel to the table through the approximate middle of the tomatoes. Lift the lid and there you have it! Use a serrated knife if your knife is dull.

Rice Noodles - Bring water to a rapid boil then turn off the heat. Submerge the noodles in the water, cover them, and set a timer for 4 minutes. Cut or bite a noodle to test for a translucent color in the center. Add more time as needed. This method gives you a longer window for perfection and less chance of overcooking them, a common error. When the noodles are soft, strain them, and run cool water over them. If you are not eating them immediately, drizzle a teaspoon or two of oil over them and toss to cover.

Peeling Shrimp - Prepare yourself with the bowl of shrimp in the sink, two bowls on the countertop, and a boning knife. Turn the cold water onto a slow stream. Cradle a shrimp in your left hand, head-end laying against the palm of your thumb, tail by your thumbnail, and feet facing your palm. Slide the tip of the knife into the pucker at the base (where the head was). Cut through the shell and halfway through the flesh, all the way down to the tail. Remove the shell (I like to keep the tail shell on) and place it in a clean bowl. Rinse the vein out of the shrimp under the running water. Place the shelled/de-veined shrimp in the second clean bowl. Another option is to use kitchen shears to cut off the shell, then slice into the flesh to de-vein. I prefer the first method as I can de-shell

and de-vein in one cut. Freeze the shrimp shells for stock or discard them.

To sous vide or not to sous vide? Cooking with a sous vide machine, or water circulator, has its pros and cons. It is excellent at creating tender and precisely cooked proteins and vegetables. The con when cooking with Reduced Oxygen Packaging or ROP (the label required for food safety practices) is that there are some potential dangers. The primary is that this method starts by removing the oxygen and vacuum sealing the food, thus creating an anaerobic, or oxygen-free environment. This allows a distinct set of pathogens to grow on the food other than the ones that emit the odor signaling spoilage. Therefore, it is important to get the right internal temperature for the correct duration of time. Also, always throw away any leftovers after 7 days, even if they smell fine.

Freezing food - When freezing food to store, restaurants often use the Individual Quick-Frozen (IQF) method. To do this, place items on a baking sheet. Make sure they are not touching. Freeze until solid, pop them off the pan, and place them into a zip-top bag before they defrost. This method keeps foods from sticking together as they freeze. It works great for freezing burger patties, meatballs, vegetables, and fruits. When freezing veggie burgers, place wax paper between each patty and put stacks of 3 in zip-top plastic bags, then pop them in the freezer. *Write reheat instructions on the plastic bag before you fill it. When freezing soup, use a large zipper lock baggie. Label and date the bag before you fill it, as the condensation will make the bag hard to write on. Place the open bag into a container. If possible, pull one edge of the bag over the lip of the container to hold it in place. Pour in the cooled liquid. Remove as much air from the bag as possible, and seal well. Place in the freezer, zipper side up if you're worried.- Jillian Forte (chef)

COOKING TRICKS
In the Church of Bacon, I have a few tenants of faith that must be followed. 1) Bake it. Either on foil or parchment paper, you will get much more consistent results from an oven than from pan-frying. 2) Bacon grease is liquid gold, so save it! You can put a coffee filter in a colander over a glass jar and tip the grease off the corner of the sheet pan, leaving you with a versatile and tasty treat. Use the oil to roast Brussel sprouts, cook

pancakes or French toast, or to make a warm vinaigrette for a tossed salad. You'll probably shake your head and wonder why you ever threw it out. - Ben Butter (line cook)

Don't buy store-bought croutons. Homemade tastes so much better, won't break your teeth, and will use up something that would normally be composted. Save ends of bread in the freezer. To use, defrost and dice. Toss the bread cubes in some oil, salt, garlic powder, and Italian seasoning and bake for 15-20 minutes at 425°. Cooking them on the stovetop over low heat also works well. Simply give them an occasional shake. - Jillian Forte (chef)

Do yourself a favor and buy kosher salt. It tastes less salty and purer than a type with added iodine. All the recipes in this book call for kosher salt. - Jillian Forte (chef)

It is true that food tastes better when cooked with love and care. Also, remember that the size and shape of veggies, the choice of temperature and speed when cooking, and the amount of stirring all affect the flavor of a dish. Bon appétit! - Kirsten Aune (prep cook)

Remember that cooking goes in one direction. You can put something back on the stove, or into the oven, but you can't un-cook it. I recommend pulling eggs off the heat before you see them at the level of doneness you're going for because the residual heat will continue to cook them for at least thirty seconds. - Ben Butter (line cook)

When putting food into a hot pan or boiling pot of water, place it gently and away from yourself so the splash goes toward the back of the stove, not toward your hands or face. - Jillian Forte (chef)

Please don't boil your vegetables, even if they come frozen! Steam them, or take a few extra minutes to toss them with some oil, salt, and pepper, and roast. Want to get crazy? Mince some garlic in there. When I was a kid, I thought I didn't like vegetables. In hindsight, what I didn't like were flavorless, boiled cellulose chunks. - Lino Rauzi (line cook)

When boiling beans, add a pinch of baking soda to the cooking water. It helps release gases that lead to flatulence. - Lyndon Ramrattan (prep cook)

If you ever burn something, call it smoked! - Jillian Forte (chef)

Never measure your ingredients over the mixing bowl or pot. If too much suddenly comes out and lands in your recipe, it's very hard to fish it out. - Rocco Salvatore (Never an employee, but always a supportive partner!)

Many recipes call for mixing the wet ingredients together separately from the dry ingredients. This is important. Adding dry spice to liquids can cause it to clump up and not mix well. Mixing all the dry ingredients, spices included, then sprinkling them over the wet ingredients creates a consistent final product. - Jillian Forte (chef)

Wet hand, dry hand. Breading with a wet ingredient like egg followed by a dry ingredient like flour or breadcrumbs can be messy. If you use the same hand for both, you are essentially breading your own fingers and making an enormous mess. To reduce the chaos, keep one hand as the "dry" hand and the other as the "wet." This method takes some getting used to, but will reduce the need to wipe your sloppy, gloppy fingers midway through the process. - Jillian Forte (chef)

One culinary trick that makes for an interesting presentation is to give height to your food. Small and tall, is the refrain in fine dining establishments. Pile the greens in the center of the plate, place the protein on the rice or potatoes so it almost stands up. Take any extra sauce, pan drippings, oils or vinegars, and drizzle them on the white space of a plate. Play with your food! Make art! - Jillian Forte (chef)

When cooking Farm to Table - Don't waste anything! Challenge yourself with what your garden has to offer in abundance, even if you don't particularly like the ingredient. At the Cafe, no zucchini is too big, or too ugly! #zucchinichallenge - Savannah Villa (baker)

Economy of Motion: It is easier and more efficient to do one action repeatedly than to move back and forth between steps. For example, if you're making more than one grilled cheese sandwich, lay out all the bread, butter all the slices so you're not picking up and putting down your knife all the time, place all the cheese. Do all the cutting at one time, or all the measuring if it's called for, etc.. - Jillian Forte (chef)

Label and date everything you put in the fridge or freezer. You may think you are going to remember what that wrapped food is, but three months later you are going to be wondering. And don't eat leftovers after 7 days. Some things don't even last that long. If you've partially eaten a dish, your bacteria is hanging out on the food. Even in the fridge, this can be a recipe for the growth of things that can make you sick. When in doubt, throw it out! - Jillian Forte (chef)

Practice, practice, practice.. be it your knife skills, different cooking methods or measurement conversions. And don't get discouraged. - Brandon Eugene (line cook)

STAY CALM! EVERYTHING WILL BE OKAY I PROMISE! Mistakes are okay. Professionals make them all the time! Just keep making 'em until you don't! - Sterling Smythe (line cook)

To all the line cooks out there... Remember, in the middle of a rush, this is not your forever, it is only your 5 minutes. Chin up and keep pushing! And of course, 2 things come for free in the kitchen, butt touches and burns - Casey Watsula (line cook)

The Cafe wasn't just another place to get coffee. It saw itself as a member of the community and made such a point to serve and support the community beyond just a good meal. This outreach and advocacy inspired me to approach the world from a similar perspective based on unity, which has helped me grow more as a human holistically. - Ramiro Figueroa (barista)

I've been a loyal neighborhood customer of the Cafe since it opened because I care about the community, food quality, and local sourcing. When I took a very part-time job in the office after I retired in 2016, my respect for Barb and Carla grew. I know firsthand that the workers are paid a decent wage and treated with respect. Restaurants are not easy places to nurture a positive work culture, but the Cafe's management succeeds in doing just that. That positive culture is reflected in the delicious food the chefs serve every single day, food that nurtures the body and the spirit. I'm happy and honored to be a small part of this wonderful local small business! - Sharla Gardner (office)

Barb and Carla are great people. They empower you, and they give you the liberty to empower everybody. They gave me a place to live in the new building. They help a lot of people. That's their MO. - Rolf Holvik (line cook)

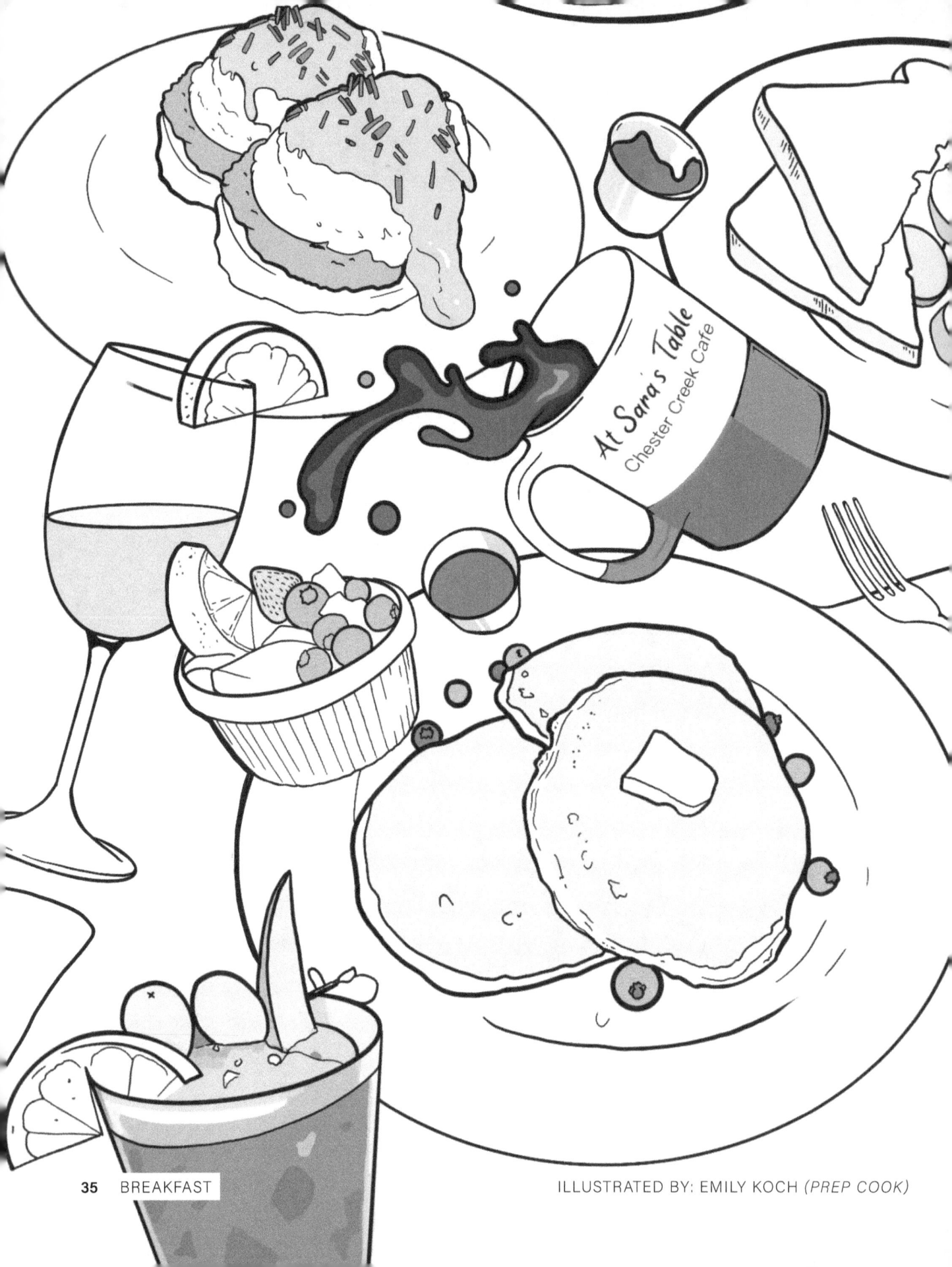

ILLUSTRATED BY: EMILY KOCH *(PREP COOK)*

breakfast

Mornings spent within At Sara's Table Chester Creek Cafe are a simple joy. On blustery winter days, the Cafe is a peaceful oasis. Early risers enjoy the smell of the wood fire crackling to life as they wrap their fingers around a hot cup of coffee and watch the sunrise over the lake. At the peak of summer, crowds flow through the doors. They nurse mimosas in the bar or sit out front on recycled plastic benches holding newspapers and conversations, waiting to be called for a table.

The foods that I've gathered in this section will help you create the satisfying feeling of a pampered morning at the restaurant. The Hippie Farm breakfast's healthy pile of sautéed vegetables, eggs, cheese, and almonds will tease your palate with each bite. The hearty Chorizo Gravy & Buttermilk Biscuits, or Original Breakfast Burrito, will fully satisfy a growling stomach. If you have a breakfast sweet tooth, try your hand at the French Toast or the Fluffy or G.F. Pancakes smothered in Maple Mascarpone and drizzled with Oatmeal Stout Beer Syrup. For an extra decadent morning, whip up a batch of Bloody Mary Mix. Every one of these dishes will start your day with love.

hippie farm

CARLA BLUMBERG 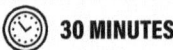 **30 MINUTES**   **SERVES 2** **VEGETARIAN** ***DAIRY-FREE**

After 17 years of working at the cafe, this dish is still my favorite to make at home! You can substitute water for wine, though the wine brings a slight acidity and sweetness to the dish. It's also a brilliant use of that quarter of a bottle that has been sitting in the fridge for who knows how long! The first 3 steps of this recipe, with the addition of spinach and white wine, will create our oft-asked-for side of veggies.

gather

cutting board, chef knife, measuring spoons, measuring cups, 12-inch sauté pan or cast iron, rubber spatula

½ medium red onion, julienned

½ medium red or green pepper, julienned

½ small zucchini, or summer squash, half-moons

1 small carrot, thin half-moons

½ cup sliced almonds, toasted

2 tsp canola oil or Butter Blend***

1 tsp fresh minced garlic

2 pinches kosher salt

2 pinches black pepper

4 eggs

2 tsp white wine or water

2 Tbsp water

½ cup shredded cheddar cheese *omit

1. Prep the ingredients. Julienne the onion and pepper to ¼-inch. Slice the zucchini into ¼-inch half-moons. Cut the carrot into half-moons slightly thinner than the zucchini. See Julienne Tip 27 and Prep Quantity 26.

2. Heat a dry sauté pan on medium-high heat. Add the almonds and toast until lightly browned. Transfer to a plate to cool.

3. Add 2 teaspoons of canola oil to the sauté pan, wait one minute. Add the onion, pepper, zucchini, and carrot. Stir occasionally for 4-5 minutes or until the onions are translucent.

4. Add the garlic, pinches of salt and pepper, and cook for one minute.

5. Pour the white wine (or water) in and mix.

6. Create a pocket in the center of the veggies by pushing everything to the sides of the pan. Crack four eggs into the space and sprinkle pinches of salt and pepper on top. If you have a 9-inch sauté pan, remove half of the veggies, create the pocket, and crack two eggs into the space. Use only half the cheese and almonds per batch. Repeat the steps 7-12 for the second batch.

7. Pour 2 tablespoons of water around the rim of the pan. Quickly cover the pan to capture the steam.

8. Baste the eggs for 3-5 minutes. Check the eggs for preferred doneness. Cook them longer for hard yokes and shorter for easy yokes. Cook the whites by gently moving them and the veggies around with a spatula.

9. When the eggs are close to done, sprinkle the cheese on top. Cover until the cheese melts.

10. Free the veggies and eggs from the pan with a spatula. Pick up the pan and slightly tip it over a plate. Slide the spatula under the eggs, gently pull the veggies and eggs onto the plate. Try to keep the eggs from flipping over.

11. Scatter the almonds on top. Serve with toast and fresh-cut fruit.

recipe tip: Basting eggs means cooking them via steam from water, sauces, or juice.

french toast batter

DIANE BAILEY & KITCHEN CREW **25 MINUTES** · **SERVES 6-8** · **VEGETARIAN** · ***DAIRY-FREE**

This French Toast is a breakfast menu classic, both sweet and satisfying. Douse it with locally sourced maple syrup from Dave Rogotzke's 'Simple Gifts,' or try our hearty house-made Oatmeal Stout Beer Syrup 48. Add a dollop of Maple Mascarpone 47, and you're nearing downright decadence. This batter recipe is simple, and works well with any bread, though the Cafe uses Cranberry-Wild Rice. The tart cranberries and the earthy flavor of the rice lend the dish its signature taste. Bonus! You can purchase loaves of our Cranberry Wild Rice Bread at the restaurant's coffee bar.

gather

bread knife, cutting board, 2 mixing bowls, liquid measuring cup, measuring spoons, whisk or immersion blender, large nonstick pan or griddle, fork, tongs

1 loaf unsliced bread or purchase Cranberry-Wild Rice bread at the Cafe

3 cups eggs, scrambled (approx. 1 dozen)

1 Tbsp vanilla extract

1 cup milk
*sub almond milk

5 Tbsp powdered sugar, plus for garnish

1 tsp ground cinnamon

1 pinch ground nutmeg

2 tsp canola oil or butter

1. Slice the bread to desired thickness using a serrated knife. At the Cafe, we cut slices a little under 1-inch thick.

2. Whisk the eggs, vanilla, and milk together in a mixing bowl until a uniform color. Note: 2% milk will lend a richness to the batter, while skim milk is healthier.

3. Stir the powdered sugar, cinnamon, and nutmeg together. Pour into the egg mixture and whisk.

4. Heat a non-stick pan over medium heat and add oil or butter to the pan. Note: Using butter will impart a rich creamy flavor, while vegetable oil is flavorless.

5. Dip each slice of bread into the batter for less than 1 minute. Dip only as many as will fit in your pan. Do not over soak the bread, as it could fall apart. Pull the bread out of the batter with tongs. Let excess batter drip back into the bowl. Note: To reduce the mess, hold a plate under the raw bread as you bring it to the pan.

6. Place the soaked bread into the hot pan and cook until golden brown, flip and repeat on the other side.

7. Repeat until the bread or batter is gone. Serve with fresh fruit, a dusting of powdered sugar, and Oatmeal Beer Stout Syrup 48!

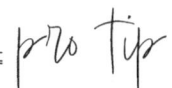

pro tip

Check that the bread is fully cooked by cutting into the center and looking inside. If you do not see the yellowish-white of the cooked egg, put a lid on the pan to capture the steam and cook it faster.

chorizo gravy

JILLIAN FORTE   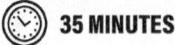 **35 MINUTES**   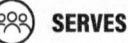 **SERVES 8**

This take on classic biscuits and gravy showcases Yker Acres' delicious pork. In 2018, I cooked this dish on stage at the State Fair. The event was hosted by Minnesota Cooks, a program created by the Minnesota Farmers Union to celebrate the partnerships between farmers and chefs. This warm golden gravy, now a customer favorite, is a perfect example of the Cafe's cuisine: local creative comfort with a twist.

gather

measuring spoons, measuring cups, heavy-bottomed pot, chef knife, cutting board, wooden-handled spoon, whisk, spatula

1 Tbsp + 1 ½ tsp fresh minced garlic

1 small yellow onion, minced

¾ cup roasted red peppers, canned, ¼-inch dice

1 ½ tsp canola oil

1 lb ground chorizo (Yker Acres)

½ lb ground pork (Yker Acres)

6 Tbsp all-purpose flour

3 cups cold chicken stock

¾ cup heavy cream

¾ tsp kosher salt

½ tsp smoked paprika, + for garnish

Buttermilk Biscuits***

½ pint cherry tomatoes, halved

1 green onion, thinly sliced

¼ bunch cilantro, stems removed

🔔 If making fresh biscuits, start those first. Once they are in the oven, make the gravy.

1. Mince the onion and garlic. Drain the red peppers and dice to 1/4-inch. Set aside.

2. Heat a heavy-bottomed pot to medium, add the oil and wait one minute. Add the minced onions, stir and cook until the onions are translucent, approx. 4 minutes.

3. Add the garlic and stir until fragrant, approx. 1 minute.

4. Add chorizo and ground pork. Use the back of a wooden spoon to break the meat into small pieces. Cook until a solid color, approx. 10 minutes.

5. Sprinkle the flour into the pot. Stir, and cook until the flour is slightly brown, 3-5 minutes Note: This is what I call a "cheater" roux.

6. Whisk in the chicken stock and heavy cream. Bring to a gentle simmer. Use a spatula to scrape any flour away from the inside edges of the pot. Whisk occasionally until the sauce bubbles and thickens.

7. Halve the cherry tomatoes. Thinly slice the green onions. Remove cilantro stems. Set aside.

8. Stir in the roasted red peppers, salt and smoked paprika. Taste for salt and spice level.

9. Pour approx. 2 cups of gravy over 2 buttermilk biscuits. Garnish with cherry tomatoes, green onions, a dash of smoked paprika, and fresh cilantro leaves!

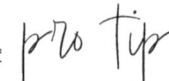

pro tip

Classic roux (a thickener for gravies and soups) is equal parts (by weight) fat and flour. To create one, melt the butter, oil or fat, then whisk in the flour. Constantly whisk or fold the flour until it turns cream-colored (blond roux) or darker brown (dark roux). Next whisk in a stock or liquid. For it to function as a thickener, the liquid must come to a bubbling simmer. However, roux will occasionally separate into oil and flour and not "work". The trick is to have either the roux or liquid be cold. In this recipe, you'll add cold stock to hot roux. When thickening a soup, you'll chill the roux and add to hot soup.

buttermilk biscuits

DIANE BAILEY 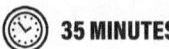 **35 MINUTES** 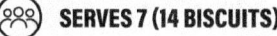 **SERVES 7 (14 BISCUITS)** **VEGETARIAN**

There are plenty of delicious biscuit recipes in the world. This one is simple. However, as with all basic recipes, the devil is in the details. Having baking experience helps, but if you have none, don't sweat it. Follow the directions closely. With time, you will notice the nuanced effects of over and under mixed dough. Good Luck!

gather

food processor, mixing bowl, circular dough/cookie cutter, baking sheet, parchment paper (optional)

3 ¾ cups all-purpose flour

2 Tbsp baking powder

⅔ tsp baking soda

1 ¼ tsp iodized salt

½ cup + 1 Tbsp + 2 tsp Crisco

1 cup cold buttermilk
(keep in the fridge until needed)

1. Heat the oven to 450°.

2. Mix the flour, baking powder, baking soda, and salt in a food processor or bowl.

3. Disperse clumps of Crisco into the flour. Lightly pulse with the processor or use a pastry knife to "chop" in the Crisco until pea-sized. It's the tiny lumps of Crisco in the flour mixture that give biscuits their fluffy texture.

4. Put the dough in a bowl and create a pocket in the center. Pour in the buttermilk. Mix with a fork. There should be wet spots and dry spots. Do not over mix, the dough should be lumpy.

5. Lay a light layer of flour on a clean dry work surface. Transfer the dough to the workspace and gently pat to about ¾-inch thick.

6. Use a circular cookie cutter to cut into biscuits. Note: Do not twist the cutter, or it will seal the edges of the biscuits and they won't rise properly. Instead, gently jiggle the cutter to loosen it from the dough.

7. Nuzzle together the remainders of dough and cut the last biscuits. Note: The second cut biscuits do not rise as well as the first, due to extra handling and subsequent squishing of the air pockets.

8. Place the biscuits onto a parchment lined baking sheet. Bake for 10-15 minutes. To ensure they are cooked in the center, open one biscuit to see if it is doughy. If the outside is golden, and the inside is raw, lower the temp on your oven and check the biscuits every 2-3 minutes.

pro tip

To get the most accurate flour measurement by volume, first fluff the flour with a spoon. Use the spoon to scoop it into a dry measuring cup. Scrape off the top with a butter knife.

original breakfast burrito with black beans & spanish sauce

 1 HOUR   **SERVES 4**   **VEGETARIAN**   ***GLUTEN-FREE**   ***DAIRY-FREE**

A much tweaked and played with concept, Breakfast Burritos have been a constant presence on the menu. This version was the longest running and featured the Black Beans and Spanish Sauce that are served over brown rice in our Peasant Bowl.

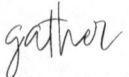 **chef's knife, cutting board, mixing bowl, measuring cups, 2 sauce pots, spatula, measuring spoons, sauté pan, mixing bowl, whisk**

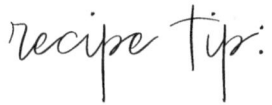 Cut all the vegetables first. There are peppers, onions and garlic in three different sections of this recipe, so it will be faster to cut them all at the start and measure when needed.

PREP

1. Cut the red and green pepper in half or use my method 28. Dice half of each pepper to ½-inch, set aside. Julienne the other halves and put into a mixing bowl.

2. Dice half of a red onion to ¼-inch, and set near the diced peppers. Julienne the other half of the onion and add to the bowl of julienned peppers.

3. Mince 4 teaspoons of garlic and set aside.

4. Slice the zucchini and carrot in half lengthwise. Cut the zucchini into half moons about ¼-inch thick. Repeat with the carrot but slightly thinner. Mix with the julienned peppers and onions. This is for burrito building.

SPANISH SAUCE

¼ cup red pepper, ½-inch dice (approx. ¼ pepper)

¼ cup green pepper, ½-inch dice (approx. ¼ pepper)

2 Tbsp red onion, ¼-inch dice (approx. ⅛ onion)

1 tsp fresh minced garlic

1 Tbsp olive oil

14.5 oz can crushed tomatoes

½ cup water

½ tsp sambal

¼ tsp kosher salt

¼ tsp black pepper

1. Heat a high-sided sauce pot on medium-high, add olive oil and wait one minute. Add ¼ cup of each diced pepper and onion. Sauté until the onions are translucent, approx. 4 minutes.

2. Add 1 teaspoon of garlic and cook for another minute.

3. Pour the can of tomatoes into the pot and stir. Add ½ cup of water to the tomato can, slosh it around and pour into the sauce.

4. Add the Sambal, salt and pepper. Stir, then lower the heat.

5. Cover the pot to prevent splattering sauce but leave it ajar so steam can escape. Let simmer for 30 minutes.

BLACK BEANS

¼ cup red pepper, ½-inch dice (about ¼ pepper)

¼ cup green pepper, ½-inch dice (about ¼ pepper)

¼ cup red onion, ¼-inch dice (about ¼ onion)

1-2 Tbsp canola oil

2 tsp fresh minced garlic

1 tsp ground cumin

2 Tbsp tomato paste

15 oz can black beans or 1 cup dried beans

¼ tsp black pepper

½ tsp kosher salt

1 Tbsp lime Juice

2-4 Tbsp water (optional)

1. Heat a sauce pot over medium-high heat, add the oil, and wait one minute. Add the remaining diced peppers and onions. Stir and cook until the onions are translucent, about 4 minutes.

2. Add 2 teaspoons of garlic, cumin, and tomato paste. Stir to combine and let cook for one minute.

3. Add the beans. You have choices. (A) Use dried beans made in advance. To cook, place the dried beans (soaked, if you had the time) into a pot or pressure cooker and add 3 cups of water and ½ teaspoon salt. Boil, cover, and lower heat to medium-low. This will take approx. 1 hour to cook. Or (B) Strain and rinse the canned beans, then add the optional water. You may need to add more salt at the end.

4. Once the beans are simmering or are completely soft, add the salt, pepper, and lime juice. Stir, then taste. Add salt or lime juice to your preference.

BURRITO BUILDING

2 tsp canola oil

½ medium red onion, julienned

½ small zucchini, julienned

1 small carrot, julienned

½ red pepper, julienned

½ green pepper, julienned

1 tsp fresh minced

garlic

8 eggs

2 pinches salt & pepper

1-2 cups shredded cheddar cheese
*omit for dairy-free

4 flour tortillas, large
*sub gluten-free

1-2 green onions
(optional)

1. Heat a large sauté pan over medium heat, add the oil, and wait one minute. Add the julienned zucchini, carrot, pepper, and onion mix. Sauté until the onions are translucent, approx. 5 minutes.

2. Crack the eggs into a mixing bowl. Whisk to an even consistency.

3. Add 1 teaspoon garlic to the sautéing vegetables and cook for one minute.

4. Pour the whisked eggs over the veggies. Add a dash of salt and pepper. Stir occasionally until the eggs are cooked to your preference.

5. Sprinkle the cheese over the eggs. Turn off the heat, cover and let the cheese melt.

6. Use a spatula to divide the eggs into four even portions.

7. Lay out the large tortillas and place a portion of eggs in the center of each one. Divide the Black Beans on top of the eggs. Fold the sides of each tortilla onto the beans, roll it up and set on a plate. Spoon the Spanish Sauce over each burrito. Garnish with extra cheese and sliced green onions.

fluffy pancakes

 35 MINUTES   **4 (8-INCH CAKES)**   **VEGETARIAN**

This is one of the few remaining, never-changed recipes at the Cafe, and the cause for an entire system update. Back in the day of handwritten paper tickets, pancakes were sold singly or as a double stack. Servers would write the word "cake" for a single, while "cakes" signified the stack of two. Well, certain people (hm hm Joe H.) had such terrible handwriting that the cooks couldn't always tell if it was 1 cake, or 2 cakes, or two people each ordering 1 cake, or 2 cakes for 2 people, or 1 cake for 1 person and 2 cakes for 2 people!! This one quirk proved so incredibly irksome that it was a big factor in the restaurant moving to a digital ordering system. We served these cakes plate sized for the adults and sporting ears and fruit faces for the kiddos.

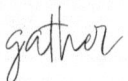 **dry measuring cups, measuring spoons, whisk, 2 mixing bowls or a stand mixer, fine-mesh strainer, liquid measuring cups, rubber spatula, large nonstick pan or griddle, ladle, flat spatula**

DRY MIX

1 ¾ cups all-purpose flour

2 Tbsp + 2 tsp white sugar

½ tsp iodized salt

1 Tbsp + ½ tsp baking powder

1 tsp baking soda

recipe tip: Close your eyes and mix the dry ingredients with your hands. The silky feeling is one of cooking's tiny pleasures.

1. Whisk or use your hands to mix all ingredients in a bowl. Note: If any ingredient looks slightly lumpy, sift it through a fine-mesh strainer to separate the hard lumps. Pulverize to dust and return to the bowl or discard.

BATTER

6 Tbsp salted butter

1 ¾ cups Dry Mix

1 ¼ cups buttermilk

1 egg

canola oil or butter

optional fillings - chocolate chips, granola, fresh fruit or toasted nuts

1. Melt the butter in the microwave.

2. Put 1 ¾ cups Dry Mix into a mixing bowl.

3. Pour the butter and buttermilk into the mixing bowl. Add the egg. Whisk until it just comes together. The batter should be lumpy, but without dry clumps. Over mixing will lead to a runny batter and flat pancakes. If the batter looks too runny, add a bit more dry mix.

4. Heat a large non-stick or well-seasoned griddle over medium heat and add 1 teaspoon of oil. Pour in a heaping ladle of the batter. Place the back of the ladle in the middle of the cake and gently spiral out to spread the pancake out into a circle. If you want to add pancake fillings, do so now.

5. When the bottom is golden brown and you see bubbles on the surface, flip the cake. Loosen all edges before flipping. If the batter isn't cooking in the center, cover the pan with a lid. This will trap the heat and cook the cake from both sides.

6. When the second side is golden brown, the cake is done. Slide it onto a plate.

7. Repeat from step 4 for the remaining batter. Serve with Maple Mascarpone 47 and real maple syrup or Oatmeal Stout Beer Syrup 48. Garnish with fruit faces for the kiddos!

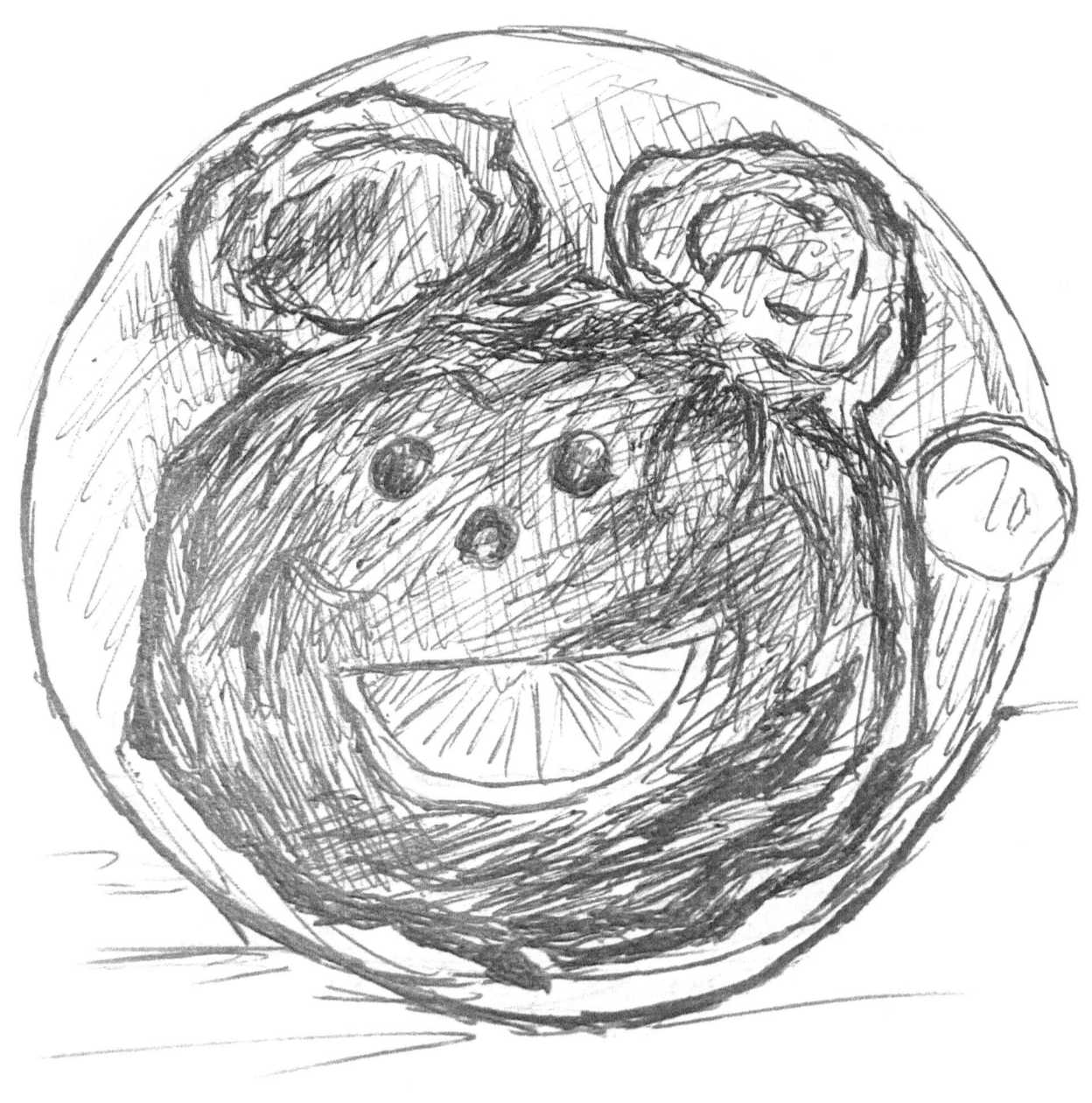

recipe tip: To create the Mickey Cakes for the kids, cook one medium-sized cake and two 2-3 inch cakes for the "ears". Arrange the face with a peeled half moon orange slice for the mouth and berries or chocolate chips for the eyes.

gluten-free pancakes

HEATHER ERICKSON   **30 MINUTES**   **12 (4-INCH CAKES)**   **DAIRY-FREE**   **GLUTEN-FREE**

As anyone with Celiac disease, or a sensitivity to gluten, knows that finding foods made without wheat flour can be difficult. Heather, our resident food allergy genius, created this pumpkin and cinnamon spiced gluten-free pancake recipe. It turned out so deliciously that they are a popular snack for the staff. Accidental "ugly" cakes never end up in the compost pile!

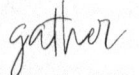 **measuring spoons, measuring cups, liquid measuring cup, 3 mixing bowls, whisk, large non-stick pan or griddle, flat spatula**

GLUTEN-FREE DRY MIX

2 ¼ cups King Arthur g.f. all-purpose flour

2 Tbsp + 2 tsp white sugar

1 ¾ tsp baking powder

⅓ tsp baking soda

½ tsp iodized salt

1. Mix all dry ingredients in a bowl. Note: If any ingredient looks lumpy, sift it through a fine-mesh strainer to separate the hard lumps. Pulverize to dust and return to the bowl or discard.

BATTER

2+ cups g.f. Dry Mix

1 tsp ground cinnamon

¼ tsp ground nutmeg

2 jumbo eggs

1 tsp vanilla extract

1 ½ cups + 2 Tbsp almond milk

6 Tbsp pumpkin puree

2 tsp canola oil

1. Put 2 cups G.F. Dry Mix into a bowl. About ½ cup will remain.

2. Add the cinnamon and nutmeg and whisk together.

3. In a separate bowl, whisk the eggs, vanilla, almond milk and pumpkin puree.

4. Pour the flour mix into the wet ingredients and whisk together. If the batter looks runny, add the reserved dry mix one tablespoon at a time until it thickens.

5. Heat a skillet or large non-stick pan over medium-high heat and add 1 teaspoon oil. Ladle approx. ¾ cup of batter into your pan. If your pan is wide enough, you can make multiple cakes at a time.

6. Once the batter bubbles in the middle, flip it over and continue to cook the other side.

7. Repeat until all the batter is cooked.

8. Freeze any leftover cakes. Reheat in a microwave, wrapped in damp paper towels.

recipe tip: Mix the wet ingredients in one bowl and the dry in a second bowl. This ensures that all ingredients, particularly the dry, fully combine in the final product. In this recipe, the cinnamon likes to ball up and not blend well with the liquids. Mixing it with flour helps it dissolve.

Barb and Carla impacted my life positively. I became endeared to Carla because I was also a cool-tempered Texan. Compared to other small business owners, she doesn't stay away from the action. She is in there doing the dirty work, even at her age. It was not uncommon to see her walking around with a screwdriver and drywall screws, or donning an apron during a particularly busy day. She has the confidence and the know-how to accomplish a wide variety of tasks. She has the ability to conceptualize what is needed, then execute it. During an illness, I had secluded myself because of covid. When I finally visited the Cafe, Carla walked right up to me and hugged me. It was the first hug in over a year. I didn't realize how much I needed that until she gave it to me. Her instinct led her to gift me what I needed. Barb and Carla had a filter that was very stringent, a standard you had to meet. Sometimes they would play good cop/bad cop. They have an unwavering philosophy of sustainability. They celebrate people of diversity and various backgrounds by giving them a chance. - Max Moen (dishwasher)

So many thoughts and memories, but overall, the ladies gave me a place to live, a place for my band to practice, and always offered me extra work when times were tough. Though we had quite a dynamic relationship, those two have huge hearts. Barb comments on my social media posts every once in a while. "Ben, you finally grew up." No, sorry Barb, still haven't. - Ben Hoffmeister (barista)

maple mascarpone

**JILLIAN FORTE &
HEATHER ERICKSON** 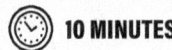 **10 MINUTES** 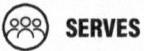 **SERVES 6** **VEGETARIAN** **GLUTEN-FREE**

I have a friend who, for years, has enjoyed brunch at the Cafe with her partner. Usually, they split a Fluffy Pancake 43, and the Hippie Farm breakfast 37. It wasn't until she was hired on with us that she realized we serve the Pancakes with Maple Mascarpone. "Jillian, I thought it was butter!" It turns out her partner loved it so much that he devoured it before she could get her hands on it! This recipe is simple but requires a little forethought. The mascarpone and cream cheese need to be at room temperature. Take them from the fridge 2 hours before mixing, and this buttery spread will go a bit more... smoothly.

gather   **measuring cups, food processor or fork, and rubber spatula**

1 cup mascarpone

½ cup cream cheese

¼ cup maple syrup

1. Blend all ingredients together. A food processor will accomplish this task in less than a minute. More than that and you will make butter! However, if you don't have a processor, a fork and spatula will work.

recipe tip: If your cheeses are cold, 20 seconds in the microwave will soften them. Do not melt the cheese, it will produce an odd texture.

> ASTCCC, was where I learned to love food. It's the place that let me explore in detail everything I had already learned and then pushed me to learn more. I owe so much of what I know about food, and where I am going with my own career, to the crew at the Cafe. People like Channie, Rolf, and Heather taught me about staying calm and having fun while cooking. Thanks, Heather and Jillian! - Brandon Eugene (line cook)

oatmeal stout beer syrup

BARB NEUBERT 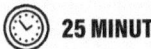 **25 MINUTES** **SERVES 16 (4 CUPS)** **VEGAN** **DAIRY-FREE**

Our locally sourced maple syrup from 'Simple Gifts' is nothing short of Northland gold! Try this variation on pure maple goodness to create a deeper, full-bodied tone. Oatmeal Stout Beer Syrup will enhance any breakfast dish that needs a bit of sweetness. It's delectable on pancakes, French toast, and oatmeal. You can even drizzle it on granola and yogurt.

gather

tall pot, liquid measuring cup, measuring spoons, rubber spatula, whisk

12 oz can oatmeal stout beer

1 ½ cups corn syrup

1 ½ cups brown sugar

¼ tsp ground cinnamon

1. Combine all ingredients except the cinnamon in a tall pot. Put on a burner over medium-high heat and stir to dissolve the sugar.

2. Bring to a boil, then immediately reduce to a low simmer.

3. Simmer on low heat, uncovered, for 15 minutes.

4. Remove from heat, then whisk in the cinnamon.

recipe tip:

Be careful. As the sugars come to a boil (over 300°), they froth and can easily boil over, causing a hot, sticky, and dangerous mess! Don't be a hot mess. Keep a close eye on this syrup.

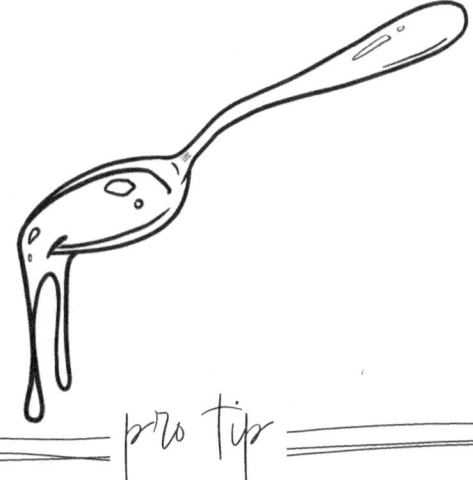

pro tip

Is my syrup done? Try the syrup test. Put a spoon into the hot syrup. When you pull it out, does the syrup separate into 2 dribbles? If yes, then it is perfect. If only one dribble forms, simmer for an additional 5 minutes.

ILLUSTRATED BY: EMILY KOCH *(PREP COOK)*

breakfast sausage

JILLIAN FORTE   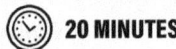 **20 MINUTES**   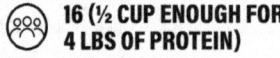 **16 (½ CUP ENOUGH FOR 4 LBS OF PROTEIN)**   **DAIRY-FREE**   **GLUTEN-FREE**   ***VEGAN**

The team and I created this recipe years ago. It started with several line cooks, creating 6 different versions of seasoning mix. We cooked up tiny batches of sausage with seasoning, then laid them out for tasting. Everyone on staff that day picked their favorite. We combined the top two winners, and, with a bit of alchemy, created one recipe that the whole crew enjoyed. The Breakfast Sausage Seasoning was a collaboration made great by an engaged and thoughtful team!

gather

measuring spoons, fork, sauté pan or cast iron, flat spatula

2 Tbsp black pepper

2 Tbsp rubbed sage

2 Tbsp dried thyme

1 Tbsp + 1 ½ tsp brown sugar

1 Tbsp kosher salt

½ tsp ground coriander

½ tsp ground fennel

⅛ tsp ground nutmeg

1 lb ground pork
*sub vegan sausage

1 tsp canola oil

1. Mix all dry ingredients together, break up any brown sugar clumps. Place in a small seal-able container.

2. Place one pound of ground pork or vegan sausage into a mixing bowl. Add 2 tablespoons of the spice blend. Mix with a fork.

3. Divide the protein into 8-10 even sized balls. Roll them in your hand to form a sphere, then flatten with the palms of your hands.

4. Heat a sauté pan over medium heat and add 1 teaspoon of oil. Place the flattened protein onto the pan and allow it to brown. Flip with a spatula and cook the other side. They are now ready to be served with your breakfast of eggs and toast!

bonus recipe

You can also cook the protein as a crumble by skipping the ball rolling step. Crumbled breakfast sausage with scrambled eggs and cheese, put into a corn tortilla with Pico de Gallo 106 creates our breakfast tacos!

bloody mary mix

HEATHER ERICKSON 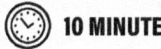 **10 MINUTES** **4 DRINKS (ABOUT 6 CUPS)**   **DAIRY-FREE**   **GLUTEN-FREE**   **VEGAN**

For some, weekend brunch would not be the same without a little "hair of the dog". This Bloody Mary Mix is earthy, rich, and salty in just the right way. No need to spice it up! Our batch size at the Cafe is about 8 times this recipe, and on hot summer mornings we sometimes have to make it twice! Most of these ingredients are probably in your kitchen, so go the extra mile and make it fresh.

gather

liquid measuring cup, measuring spoons, mixing bowl, whisk, saucer, 4 pint glasses

46 oz can V8, organic if possible

⅔ cup dill pickle juice

1 tsp black pepper

1 tsp ground mustard powder

1 tsp celery salt

½ tsp garlic powder

1 Tbsp +1 tsp white vinegar

2 tsp horseradish

1 tsp Sriracha

½ lemon, juiced

1+ Tbsp celery salt (optional garnish)

8 oz local vodka

1. Whisk all ingredients together except the last tablespoon of celery salt and vodka.

2. Put 1 Tbsp celery salt onto a saucer. Wet the rims of 4 pint glasses. One at a time, place the rims into the salt and twist the cup.

3. Pour 2 ounces of your favorite vodka in each pint glass. Fill the glass halfway with ice cubes and top off with about 1 ½ cups of Bloody Mary mix.

4. Garnish the drink with any or all of the following; lemon wedge, celery stick, olives, beef stick, cheese cubes and a snit of your favorite beer. You know the drill!

"Bartending at the Cafe was such a warm experience; the regulars, Service Industry Night folks, and getting to make cocktails for my coworkers all made my time there so memorable." - Anna Brown (bartender)

"It was relaxed and such a great room. It felt like an old bar that was kept in good condition over the years." - Jesse Hoheisel (bartender)

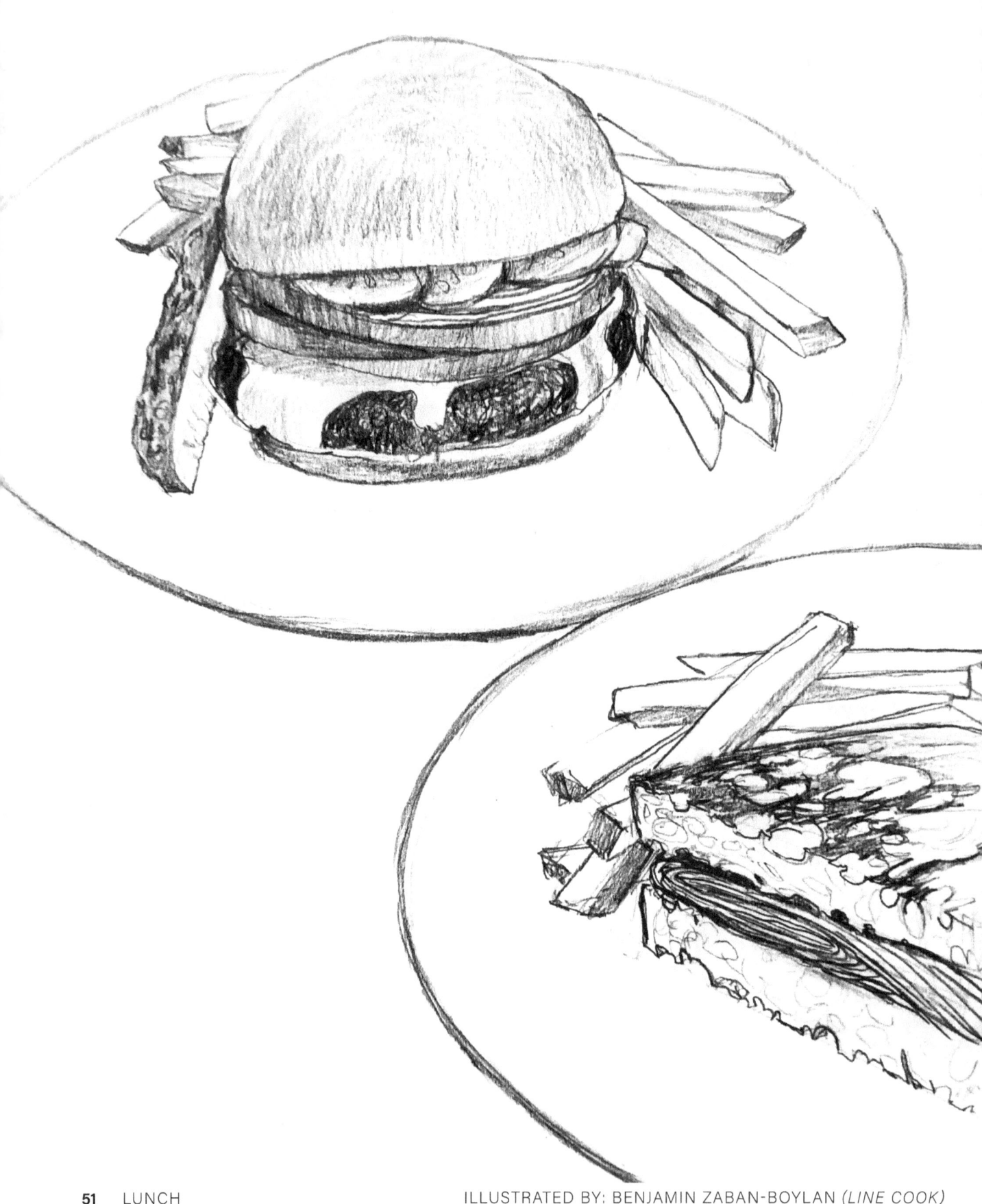

ILLUSTRATED BY: BENJAMIN ZABAN-BOYLAN *(LINE COOK)*

lunch

"Let's do lunch!" I think of lunch as community-building time, a time to weave social fabric over a shared meal. The Cafe can be a very busy scene during the lunch hour. Customers cover the tables with notebooks and gift bags intermingled with steaming soups, aromatic burgers, and glasses of cold lemonade. To gather for a meal is to create a magic that binds. Even amidst our busy lives, lunch is a daily testament to connecting!

Due to the quick pace of serving lunch at the Cafe, many of the dishes in this section can be prepared in advance. The Okonomiyaki, Quinoa Veggie Burger, and Seafood Burger require prep time, but can then be served up with little fuss. The Baja Slaw for the Colorful Baja Fish Tacos and Bulgogi Tacos are easily assembled, but they taste best when allowed to marinate for 12-24 hours. The Yucatan Carnitas meat has a long, slow simmer time, but can be chilled and reheated quickly. Make the Tabbouleh and Hummus in advance. You'll need only to set them on the table at mealtime with cut veggies or Fresh Pita Bread 80. The Kung Fu Noodles and Deluxe Grilled Cheese are quick and wallop the mouth with flavor! Prep in advance and focus your lunch hour on connecting with companions.

okonomiyaki & spicy vegan aioli

JILLIAN FORTE & HEATHER ERICKSON   🕐 **1 HOUR & 10 MINUTES**   👥 **SERVES 4**   **GLUTEN-FREE**   **VEGAN**

The creation of this very popular dish has an interesting backstory. While reading a foodie magazine, I ran across this list of "Top 20 Things Chefs put on Menus that Confuse Customers." I knew 18 off the list, had heard of another, but the last was a complete mystery. I didn't even know how to pronounce it! As a culinarily curious chef, I jumped into the research. Okonomiyaki is a popular street pancake in Japan. It's made with vegetables and eggs and covered in sauces and garnishes. I didn't know if the dish would fly with Midwestern palates, but I knew dietary restraints make for adventurous eaters, so I created a version of Okonomiyaki that was vegan and gluten-free. This savory pancake is more crumbly than the traditional version, but it tastes just as scrumptious and our customers love it.

Vegans, I know you love creamy-textured, fatty foods! If you haven't made your own mayonnaise, today is the day. It's easy, and once you have the base, you can spice it and spike it any way you desire. Honestly though, the flavor profile presented here is exceptional on lots of different dishes. Try it on Roasted Root Vegetables 99, a Buddha Bowl 83, or as a spread on just about any sandwich.

gather **chef knife and cutting board, liquid measuring cup, measuring spoons, one large and one small mixing bowl, vegetable peeler, tongs, large mixing spoon, flat spatula, sauté pan, blender**

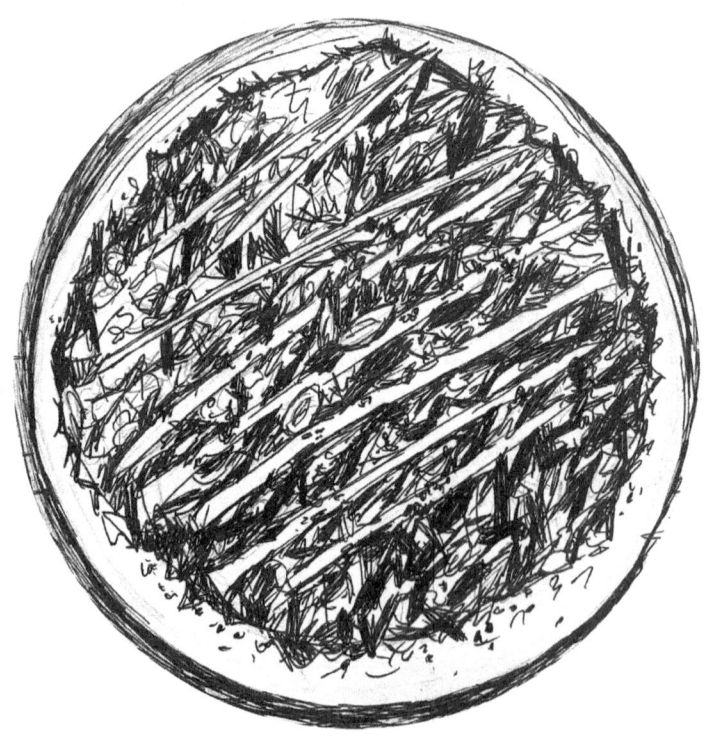

ILLUSTRATED BY: MELISSA WEISSER (*SERVER*)

OKONOMIYAKI PREP

1 cup red pepper, julienned (approx. ½)

2+ cups green cabbage, sliced (approx. ¼ head)

4 green onions, sliced, divided

½ cup carrot, shredded (approx. 1)

1⅓ cups shiitake caps, sliced (approx. 2- 5oz containers)

¾ tsp fresh minced ginger

2 cups shredded hash browns (store-bought)

½ cup crumbled tofu

1 Tbsp + 1 tsp g.f. tamari, or soy sauce

½ tsp rice vinegar

¼ cup water

3 Tbsp corn starch

1 Tbsp nori, crumbled (approx. ½ sheet)

6 Tbsp oat flour or ground flax

6 Tbsp garbanzo bean flour, aka cici bean or chickpea flour

2 Tbsp nutritional yeast, preferably flakes

½ tsp kosher salt

1-3 tsp canola oil

1 cup Spicy Vegan Aioli or Spicy Aioli

1⅓ cups Matt's Kimchi 109 or store-bought

½ bunch cilantro, garnish

1. Prep the ingredients. As you cut each vegetable, place it together in a large mixing bowl. Julienne half a red pepper into ⅛-inch thick strips. See Julienne Tip 27. Slice the cabbage to ⅛-inch or thinner. Slice green onions as thin as possible, and set aside ¼ cup for garnish. Peel, then shred ½ cup carrot on a box grater. De-stem the shiitakes, discard the stems (or save for stock). Slice the caps to ¼ - ⅛-inch. Peel then mince the ginger until you get ¾ teaspoon. See Pro Tip below. De-stem the cilantro leaves, and set them aside for garnish.

2. Place the hash browns in the bowl on top of the veggies.

3. Crumble, then measure the tofu. Pour half the tamari on the tofu and half on the hash browns. Mix the tofu and tamari together and add to the bowl.

4. Sprinkle the rice vinegar over the veggies.

5. Stir the water and the cornstarch together until milky colored. Pour over the veggies.

6. Toast and crumble the nori. Use tongs to pass the nori sheet over the flames of your gas burner, or put it in a hot sauté pan until it blisters, flipping as necessary. It will crumble easily by hand. If you're short on time, skip the toasting. However, you will need to cut it into ½-inch or smaller pieces.

7. Mix the nori, flours, nutritional yeast, and salt in a mixing bowl, then sprinkle over the veggie mix. See Wet/Dry Tip 32.

8. Mix all the ingredients until there are no wet or dry spots or clumps. Note: This mixture keeps for about 3-4 days in the fridge, after which the veggies will weep and become soggy.

🔔 If making the Vegan Aioli, do so now.

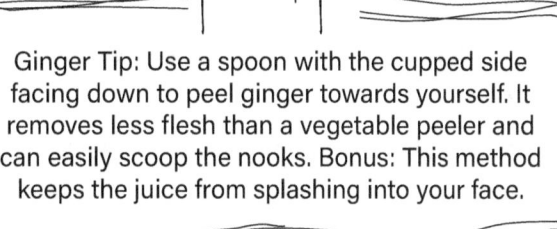

pro tip

Ginger Tip: Use a spoon with the cupped side facing down to peel ginger towards yourself. It removes less flesh than a vegetable peeler and can easily scoop the nooks. Bonus: This method keeps the juice from splashing into your face.

VEGAN AIOLI

½ cup soy milk or almond milk

2 ½ tsp cider vinegar

¼ tsp rice vinegar

½ fresh lemon, juiced

1 tsp kosher salt

⅛ tsp granulated garlic

2 ½ tsp dijon mustard

½ cup canola oil

½ cup olive oil

1. Put the soy milk, both kinds of vinegar, lemon juice, salt, garlic, and dijon into a blender or food processor.

2. Measure the oils in a liquid measuring cup.

3. Turn the blender to medium speed and drizzle the oil in from above. As the aioli thickens, gradually increase the pouring speed. If the oil is accumulating faster than it is incorporated, slow down or stop until it has caught up. Note: You can whisk the aioli, though it will require a bit of elbow grease.

SPICY VEGAN AIOLI

1 ½ cups vegan aioli or mayonnaise

1 Tbsp + 2 ½ tsp sambal

1 ½ tsp Sriracha

1 tsp g.f. tamari, or soy

1. Put the vegan aioli into a blender or mixing bowl.

2. Process or whisk the sambal, Sriracha, and tamari until combined.

COOKING THE OKONOMIYAKI

1. Heat a non-stick sauté pan over medium-high heat (a curved edge pan will make for easier flipping). Add 1 teaspoon oil and wait one minute.

2. Add about 2-3 cups of the mix into the pan, to a thickness of 1-inch. The mixture should sizzle. Immediately jiggle the pan to prevent sticking. Flatten and compact the Oki with a spatula.

3. Fry until the bottom is crispy and brown, approx. 4-6 minutes.

4. Flip and repeat. If you are not confident in your flipping skills, use a spatula to divide the Oko into four sections, then flip each one. You can reshape the pieces into a pancake.

5. Once crispy on the second side, slide the pancake onto your plate. Repeat from step 2 until all the mix is gone.

6. Garnish each cake with a lattice of Spicy Vegan Aioli, ⅓ cup kimchi, cilantro leaves, and reserved green onions.

I absolutely enjoyed working for the ladies! It was a seminal time in my life. I learned a lot and made lifelong friends! Though I was hired as a barista and server, I eventually became the front-of-house manager. In that capacity, I learned every job in the Cafe, from the dish pit to the line, to menu design, and scheduling. Some of my favorite shifts were prep cooking with Jillian and Christopher. I miss those days.
- Sarah Runholt-Farrell (FOH manager)

"I remember Toni Bologna hid in the fridge in the coffee bar. They had cleaned it, so everything was out of it. I came up not knowing any of this and I opened up the cooler and she was standing in the fridge. It scared the Hell out of me. You know, you just don't expect to see a person standing in a refrigerator."
-Diane Bailey (baker)

quinoa veggie burger

HEATHER ERICKSON **2 HOURS (+2-24 HOURS)** **SERVES 12-13**   **GLUTEN-FREE**   **DAIRY-FREE**   **VEGAN**

Our food allergy specialist, Heather, created this gluten-free veggie burger. The quinoa adds a nice chewy texture, while all the fresh veggies keep the nutritional value high. This process is a bit messy and time-consuming, but it's worth it. You will form and par-bake the patties and can freeze any extras. The longer prep time makes for quick meals in the future. From freezer to plate in 30-40 minutes!

2-24 hours ahead: Bake two potatoes at 450° for 40 minutes or until soft inside. Cool completely, approx. 2-24 hours.

gather **pot and lid, chef knife, cutting board, 3 mixing bowls, zester, food processor or potato masher, rubber spatula, baking sheet, plastic lid, and plastic wrap (optional)**

1 ½ cups baked and cooled russet potatoes (approx. 2)

1 cup quinoa

2 ½ cups water, divided

1 medium green pepper, ¼-inch dice

1 medium red pepper, ¼-inch dice

1 small yellow onion, ¼-inch dice

½ small jalapeño, minced

½ cup fresh minced parsley (approx. ½ bunch)

½ cup fresh minced cilantro (approx. ⅔ bunch)

¼ cup fresh minced garlic (approx. 12 cloves)

½ fresh lemon, zest, and juice

15 oz can black beans, drained

¼ cup tahini

8 oz tempeh, crumbled

1 Tbsp Sriracha

2 Tbsp curry powder

2 Tbsp ground cumin

1 Tbsp +1 ½ tsp iodized salt

2 cups rice flour, brown or white

1-2 tsp canola oil or pan spray

1. Rinse the quinoa in a fine-mesh strainer, and put it into a pot. Add 2 cups of water and bring to a boil. Cover and lower the heat to a simmer. Set a timer for 15 minutes.

2. Cut each vegetable, then place them together in a large mixing bowl. Dice the peppers and onion to ¼ -inch or smaller. Remove the seeds from the jalapeño (keep them, if you want spicier burgers) and mince. Rinse the herbs and shake dry. De-stem the parsley, set leaves aside, and discard the stems (or save for stock). Remove and discard thick cilantro stems. Mince each herb, and add to the bowl. Mince the garlic and add to the bowl.

3. Check the quinoa for white specs. If visible, stir, replace the lid but turn off the heat. The steam will finish the cooking process. Once fully cooked, transfer to a plate and chill in the fridge.

4. Zest half the lemon into the bowl. Halve the lemon and juice one half into the bowl. See Citrus Juicing Tip 27.

5. Peel, rough chop, and measure 1 ½ cups of the cooled baked potato.

6. Put potatoes into a food processor or a wide-bottomed bowl. Add half of the black beans, all the tahini, and ½ cup of water. Pulse or mash (with a potato masher) scraping down the sides as needed until you create a uniform paste. This paste is the binder. Add it and the remaining whole black beans to the mixing bowl.

7. Crumble or mince the tempeh and add to the bowl.

8. Add the cooled quinoa and Sriracha.

9. Combine the curry, cumin, salt, and flour in a clean bowl. Mix and sprinkle over the mixture.

10. Heat the oven to 400° (before your hands get dirty).

11. Use bare hands, wear disposable gloves, or use a large metal spoon to fully combine the mixture.

12. Form 12-13 patties. You can "eyeball" this to approximately the same size and free-style the shape. Or you can use the Cafe Tip below for our ingenious, efficient but peculiar method.

13. Par-bake the patties on a greased baking sheet for 30-35 minutes. Flip once at the 15-minute mark.

14. For immediate eating, toss the patties on the grill or in a sauté pan with a little oil and cook for 5-10 minutes. Freeze extra burgers using the Freezing Tip 30. Note: If preparing the burger from frozen, thaw for 15-25 minutes before cooking.

recipe Tip: Use a 4-5 oz ice cream scoop to form consistent-sized balls. Find a jar lid that is about 4-inches wide and about ½ -inch deep (large pickle jar or peanut butter lid). Lay the lid on the table so the cupped side is up. Place a sheet of plastic wrap over it, with about 3-inches hanging off each end. Fit the plastic to the lid's interior and wrap the plastic flaps onto the back. Oil the plastic inside the lid and off you go. Pat a ball of the mixture firmly inside the lid, flip over, press down, lift the lid, and Voila' a perfectly shaped patty! Thanks to Rigs for this creative idea.

pro tip

Use a reusable coffee filter to rinse the quinoa. The mesh is so fine the grains won't slip through.

Working at Chester Creek Cafe was far more than a job. Besides allowing me the opportunity to learn skills, the experience opened the door to friendships and connections. The women of ASTCCC are some of the strongest leaders I have ever had the chance to work with. I am honored to have been a small part of such an amazing team and am forever grateful for the opportunity. - Jon Otis (line cook)

lemony tabbouleh

 50 MINUTES   **4 (1 CUP PORTIONS)**   **VEGAN**   **VEGETARIAN**   **DAIRY-FREE**

Do you miss the Mediterranean plate? Don't we all! This tabbouleh is a refreshing, flavorful, mouth-happy dish. As always, use high-quality ingredients. Choose an olive oil that tastes good to you. Squeeze fresh lemons. Add a sprinkle of feta cheese, olives, or pepperoncini if making the dish into a full meal. This recipe requires a lot of chopping. I like to think of it as an excellent opportunity to practice mindfulness.

gather

small pot and cover, chef knife, cutting board, mixing bowl, mixing spoon or spatula, measuring spoons and cups, vegetable peeler

1 cup water

1 pinch kosher salt

½ tsp dried mint or 1 tsp fresh minced mint

½ cup bulgar wheat

2 Tbsp fresh minced mint

3 Tbsp fresh minced parsley (approx. ¼ bunch)

¼ cup green onions, minced (approx. 2-3)

1½ cups cucumber, ¼-inch dice (approx. 1)

2 cups tomatoes, ½-inch dice (approx. 2 large or 3-5 plum)

1+ tsp fresh minced garlic

¼ cup extra virgin olive oil

2+ Tbsp lemon juice (approx. 1)

1. Boil 1 cup of water in a small pot. Add the salt, ½ teaspoon dried mint (or 1 teaspoon fresh minced mint), and bulgar. Cover and turn off the heat. Steam for 15-20 minutes. Cool bulgar on a plate in the fridge.

2. De-stem and mince the mint and parsley. Mince the green onions. Place all in a medium-sized mixing bowl.

3. Peel, de-seed (use a spoon), and dice the cucumber to ¼-inch. Add to the mixing bowl. Note: English cucumbers, usually shrink-wrapped in plastic, have very tender and edible skin. They need to be washed, not peeled.

4. Slice the tomatoes in half and de-seed them by pushing your fingers into each spot with seeds. Dice to approximately ½ - ¼-inch and add to the bowl. The knife won't slice the tomato? See Tomato Tip 29.

5. Add the garlic, olive oil, lemon juice, and cooled bulgar. Mix well.

6. Taste for salt, lemon, and garlic. Adjust to your preference.

pro tip

Keep a bowl for compost scraps next to your workstation to collect the juicy tomato seeds, stems, and skins. This makes cleaning up a lot more efficient.

classic hummus

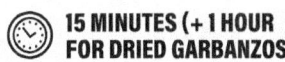 15 MINUTES (+ 1 HOUR FOR DRIED GARBANZOS)   4 (½ CUP SERVINGS)   **GLUTEN-FREE**   **VEGAN**   **DAIRY-FREE**

The nutty flavor of protein-rich chickpeas makes hummus a staple in many vegetarian households. This recipe is from the Cafe's memorable Mediterranean plate. Hummus is flavorful on its own, as a dip, or smeared on a sandwich. I like a light layer of hummus and fresh tomatoes inside grilled cheese. You can use canned garbanzo beans in this recipe; however, if you boil dried beans, reserve the leftover water. The gelatinous liquid is called aquafaba and is a vegan substitute for eggs.

gather

pot or pressure cooker (for cooking garbanzos), measuring cups and spoons, food processor, kitchen blender or immersion blender, rubber spatula

6 oz dried garbanzo beans or 15 oz can

3 Tbsp lemon juice

2 Tbsp tahini

2 Tbsp extra virgin olive oil, plus for garnish

¾ tsp sesame oil

1 Tbsp fresh minced garlic

1 ¼ tsp ground cumin

¾ tsp kosher salt

1 pinch cayenne powder

2 Tbsp water

2 dashes paprika (optional garnish)

1 Tbsp fresh minced parsley (optional garnish)

1. If using dried garbanzo beans, boil until soft. Strain and cool (reserve the liquid for aquafaba). If using canned beans, drain the liquid. Pro Tip: Once the cooked garbanzo beans are cool, you can remove loose skins from the beans. This lends a creamier texture; however, it's unnecessary and doesn't change the flavor.

2. If using an immersion blender, put all the ingredients into a tall-sided bowl and blend until smooth. You may need to scrape down the sides of the bowl. Move to step 5.

3. If using a food processor or blender, put half of the garbanzo beans, the lemon juice, and tahini into the container. Puree until smooth. If the blades won't pull the beans in, stop the machine, scrape down the sides and add 1-2 tablespoons water. Scoop the pureed beans from the machine into a mixing bowl.

4. Put the remaining beans in the food processor along with the oils, garlic, and spices. Puree until smooth. Scrape down the sides and add the remaining water if necessary. Note: If you like thick hummus, don't add all the water. If you like a dip and scoop-able hummus, add all the water and possibly a bit more. Combine the two batches of beans in the mixing bowl.

5. Add salt and garlic to your preference. Serve with a drizzle of extra virgin olive oil, a dash of paprika, and minced parsley.

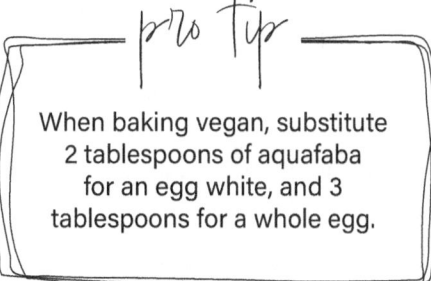
pro tip
When baking vegan, substitute 2 tablespoons of aquafaba for an egg white, and 3 tablespoons for a whole egg.

ham & gouda melt, honey mustard & caramelized onions

PETER RAVINSKI, JILLIAN FORTE, & MICAH NEWMAN   **1 HOUR**   **SERVES 2**   ***GLUTEN-FREE**

This sandwich melt, a nice riff on a classic ham and cheese, held a place on the Cafe menu for nearly a decade. Make a double batch of caramelized onions. They are fabulous in pasta, omelets, or soup. The honey mustard is so versatile it will probably become a staple condiment in your kitchen.

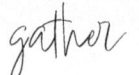 **chef knife, cutting board, tongs, rondeau or cast iron, mixing bowl, measuring cups and spoons, whisk, metal spatula, sauté pan**

CARAMELIZED ONIONS

3 large white onions

1-2 Tbsp salted butter

¼ tsp kosher salt

1 tsp sherry or red wine

1 pinch white sugar
(optional)

1. Julienne the onions. See Julienne Tips 27.

2. Melt the butter in a heavy-bottomed rondeau pan or cast iron on medium heat. See Pan Types illustration 21. Put the onions in the pan. Stir and sweat until translucent, approx, 10 minutes.

3. Stir in the salt and lower the heat.

4. Over the next hour, occasionally stir the onions, but mostly leave them alone. Caramelizing takes patience and a watchful eye. The longer you babysit this process, the darker and sweeter your onions will become. Watch the onions cook down and darken. Smell them sweeten as the sugars caramelize. Listen to the pan. It should be quiet. If you hear sizzling, stir, or lower the heat. When you notice the sides of the pan are brown, use the onions to rub this flavor off the pan and back into the onions. That sticky golden brown is caramelized sugar! If your onions smell burned or look black at any point, turn off the heat. All is not lost. Pour in the sherry or a splash of water, cover the pan and let them sit for 3-5 minutes. This allows the wine to steam the onions and de-glaze the pan, pulling the sugars back into the onions. Stir. You can turn the heat back on at a lower temperature and keep cooking.

   🔔 While the onions are cooking, start the Honey Mustard.

5. Once you feel done, at whichever color gradient you have accomplished, taste a small bite of the onions. If you'd like them sweeter, add a pinch of sugar and stir. This isn't cheating, it's just a trick!

6. Use on the Ham & Gouda Melt or put in an uncovered container in the fridge to cool. Once cold, cover tightly. They'll keep for about a week.

HONEY MUSTARD

2 Tbsp sour cream

2 Tbsp mayonnaise
(Hellman's)

1 Tbsp dijon mustard

1 Tbsp whole grain mustard

1 Tbsp honey

¾ tsp yellow mustard

¾ tsp red wine vinegar

1. Whisk all ingredients in a mixing bowl. Note: Store extra in a tightly sealed, labeled container in the fridge for up to 2 weeks.

SANDWICH

1 Tbsp salted butter

4 slices whole-wheat bread *sub g.f.

8 oz shaved ham

4 slices smoked gouda
(Eichten's)

¼ cup Caramelized Onions

¼ cup Honey Mustard

1. Spread the butter on one side of each slice of bread.

2. Smear the dry side with 1-2 tablespoons of Honey Mustard. Layer a slice of gouda, 4 oz of ham, 2 tablespoons of caramelized onions, and another slice of gouda, followed by the last slice of bread.

3. Place both sandwiches in a cold pan and heat the pan to medium heat. Cook until golden. Flip the sandwiches and repeat on the other side.

pro tip

Starting with a cold pan, when making grilled cheese or melts, allows the heat to flow through the bread and melt the cheese as it comes up to temperature. Starting with a hot pan browns the bread without melting the cheese.

pro tip

In a hurry? Heat the pan to medium-high. Butter the bread, and add the honey mustard and cheese to all slices. Place in the pan and let the cheese melt. Mound the ham in the pan, off to the side (or in a second pan), place the onions on top, and heat until steaming. Flip as needed. Use a spatula to slide the hot ham and onions onto the cheese-covered bread and put the sandwich together.

kung fu noodle bowl

BRUCE WALLIS **20 MINUTES** **SERVES 4**   **GLUTEN-FREE**   **VEGAN**   **DAIRY-FREE**

These noodles were a staff after-shift meal favorite. They make a quick and light lunch, or an excellent side with Beef Bulgogi 70, or Braised Beef Short Ribs 85. The zingy ginger, sharp green onions, and sweet carrot sticks pack a powerful flavor punch, thus their name, Kung Fu!

gather   **pot, chef knife, cutting board, box grater, measuring cups and spoons, strainer, mixing bowl**

¾ - 1 cup green onions, sliced (approx. 7-9)

1 cup matchstick carrots (store-bought or shredded)

4 Tbsp fresh minced ginger

3 Tbsp canola oil, divided

1 ½ tsp g.f. tamari, or soy sauce

¾ tsp sherry vinegar

1 tsp kosher salt

14 oz bag rice sticks, thin

2 tsp sesame oil (dark-colored)

2 Tbsp sambal (optional)

4 lime wedges (optional)

1. Boil 2-3 quarts of water in the pot.

2. Thinly slice the green onions in their entirety, green and white parts, minus the fringe. (This is an excellent test of your knife's sharpness.) Put in a medium-sized mixing bowl.

3. Add the carrot, ginger, 2 tablespoons plus 1 teaspoon canola oil, tamari, vinegar, and salt. Mix well and set aside.

4. Cook the rice noodles. You can follow the instructions on the back of the package or see Rice Noodle Tip 29. Once the noodles are soft but not falling apart, strain and run under cold water. While still in the strainer, pour 1-2 teaspoons of canola or sesame oil over the noodles, and mix until covered.

5. Divide the noodles into 4-5 plates. Place approx. ¼ cup of the Kung Fu slaw on top of each pile of noodles. Serve with tamari, sambal, and lime wedges.

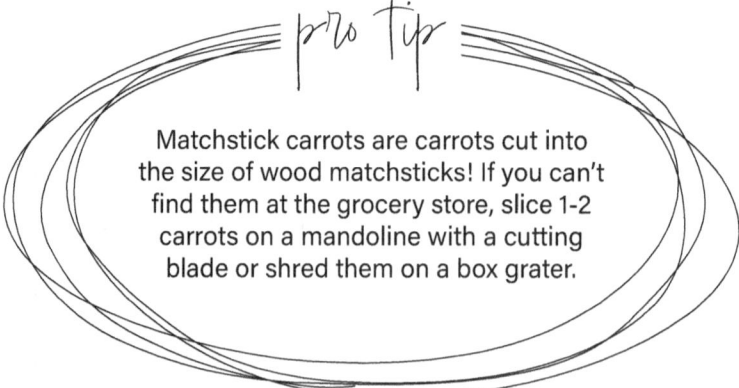

pro tip

Matchstick carrots are carrots cut into the size of wood matchsticks! If you can't find them at the grocery store, slice 1-2 carrots on a mandoline with a cutting blade or shred them on a box grater.

deluxe grilled cheese

JILLIAN FORTE   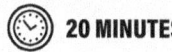 **20 MINUTES**   **SERVES 4-5**   ***GLUTEN-FREE**

Calling all blue cheese lovers! This mouth-watering, decadent, grilled cheese is for you. Apple juice is the recipe's secret ingredient. It adds a sweetness that complements and cuts the pungency of the blue and brie cheeses. A quality blue cheese will make all the difference, so pass over the tubs of crumbled at the store, and buy a true wedge from your favorite cheesemonger. We serve this sandwich with Tomato Bisque 147. It also pairs well with fresh apple slaw.

gather

food processor or bowl and wooden spoon, measuring cups and spoons, sauté pan, flat spatula, serrated knife, cutting board

¼ cup crumbled blue cheese

2 Tbsp brie, most of the rind removed

¼ cup chevre

1 Tbsp apple juice

6 Tbsp shredded Parmesan

4 1 oz Havarti slices
(enough to cover 4 slices of bread)

4 1 oz cheddar slices
(enough to cover 4 slices of bread)

2 Tbsp salted butter

1 loaf whole-grain bread
*sub g.f. bread

1. Blend the blue cheese, brie, chevre, apple juice, and Parmesan in the food processor for about 1 minute or until everything is incorporated. Sans food processor, use a blender to first crumble the Parmesan. Add the blue cheese, brie, and apple juice and blend. Scoop into a bowl, add the chevre and mix well with a wooden spoon or fork.

2. Smear butter on one side of 8-10 slices of bread. Lay a slice of Havarti and cheddar on half the slices of bread. On the other half smear about ¼-⅓ cup of the cheese blend. Put the two halves together.

3. Place the sandwiches in a cold sauté pan. Turn the heat to medium-low. Note: Slow and steady heat will give the cheese time to melt before the bread gets too dark. Once the bottom side is golden brown, flip the sandwich and continue cooking. If you are in a hurry, keep the sandwich open, cook each side separately, then place it together once the cheese is melted.

4. Remove the cooked sandwiches to a cutting board. Cut the sandwiches in half using a serrated knife so the cheese doesn't ooze out.

> *It was a great learning experience that enabled me to bake almost anything, let alone make it gluten-free and/or vegan without sacrificing taste and texture. Being able to provide a tasty treat for someone with a food allergy was, and still is, very rewarding. Food allergies don't have to feel like a complete punishment anymore.*
> — *Savannah Villa (baker)*

seafood burger & lime caper aioli

PETER RAVINSKI **45 MINUTES** **SERVES 6**   **DAIRY-FREE**   ***GLUTEN-FREE**

At home, I happily freeze leftover fish, knowing I'll get to use it for Seafood Burgers. Stick with the recipe's prescribed proportion, but feel free to substitute any type of fish—walleye for the whitefish, shrimp for the crab, etc. The lime caper aioli is my "go-to" sauce for fish. It's similar to a tartar sauce in consistency, but the lime and caper give it more zing and depth.

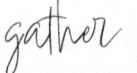 **pot, chef knife, and cutting board, measuring spoons and cups, mixing bowl, sauté pan, flat spatula, mixing spoon**

SEAFOOD BURGER

1 cup cooked salmon

2 ¼ cups cooked white fish

1 ¼ cup canned crab

½ cup red onion, ¼-inch dice (approx. ¼)

½ cup red pepper, ¼-inch dice (approx. ½)

2 Tbsp minced green onion (approx. 1)

1 tsp fresh minced garlic

½ cup corn kernels

¼ cup mayonnaise (Hellman's)

1 Tbsp dijon mustard

½ tsp Worcestershire sauce

1 ½ tsp lemon juice

1 egg

1 Tbsp Old Bay seasoning

¼ tsp kosher salt

½-1 cup bread crumbs *sub g.f. bread

1 Tbsp canola oil

6 burger buns *sub g.f. buns

1. Place the cooked seafood in a large mixing bowl. Remove any skin or bones. If using shrimp, chop it into ¼-inch pieces.

2. Dice the red onion and red pepper to ¼ -inch. Mince the green onion and garlic. Add to the mixing bowl.

3. Add the corn, mayonnaise, mustard, Worcestershire, lemon juice, and egg to the bowl.

4. Sprinkle in the Old Bay and salt.

5. Add ½ cup of breadcrumbs to the bowl. Mix, combining with a spoon, spatula, or hands. Try not to mash the fish. Half-inch-sized pieces of fish in the burger are nice, a pulpy glop is not. If the mix does not stick together when compacted in your hand, add more bread crumbs.

6. Hand form the patties to 1-inch thick and the approximate width of the burger buns.

7. Heat a sauté pan to medium and add 1 teaspoon of canola oil. Place the patties in the pan. Cook until golden brown. Flip and continue cooking.

   🔔 If making the Lime Caper aioli, start that while the burgers are cooking.

8. Place the burgers in the buns with about 2 tablespoons of aioli and any fixings you enjoy.

LIME CAPER AIOLI

2 Tbsp capers, minced

1 tsp fresh minced tarragon or basil

1 cup mayonnaise
(Hellman's)

1 Tbsp + 1 ½ tsp lime juice

1 pinch granulated garlic

1 dash kosher salt

1 dash black pepper

1. Mince the capers and tarragon. Place in a small mixing bowl.

2. Add the mayonnaise, lime juice, granulated garlic, salt, and pepper and mix well. Store extras in a tightly sealed, labeled container in the fridge for up to 2 weeks.

pro tip

To poach raw fish, gently simmer a pot of water or fish stock. Add 1 tablespoon salt and a teaspoon of Old Bay. Submerge the uncooked, defrosted seafood. Simmer on low for approx. 5-7 minutes. Check the inside of the fish for a solid, not opaque color. Strain from the water and place in the fridge to cool.

My time at ASTCCC was the longest I ever worked at a restaurant, 7 years, all in front-of-the-house positions. When I moved away, I realized how much Barb and Carla cared, and also that the Cafe was organized and clean. My introduction to different worldly cuisines, foods, and terms expanded 10 fold while I was there. I never knew aioli's, remoulade, bibimbap, curry, even ramekins, or Cubano coffees where cinnamon and sugar are mixed with the espresso grounds or smoothie bases where you freeze the fruit instead of using ice. I learned and grew a lot there. - Faith Woodruff (FOH manager)

colorful baja fish tacos

BRUCE WALLIS   **3 HOURS**   **SERVES 4 (3 TACOS EACH)**   **DAIRY-FREE**   **GLUTEN-FREE**

This refreshingly bright recipe makes a yummy summer taco that leaves me feeling fueled and ready for adventure. The tacos are easy to make, though they require some planning. The slaw should marinate for at least 2 hours and up to 2 days. For a quick, guest-pleasing, dinner party, serve with Arroz Verde 115, cold lager, or chilled wine.

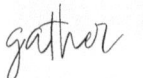

chef knife, cutting board, large and small mixing bowls, measuring spoons and cups, whisk, box grater, small plate, mandoline slicer (if available), aluminum foil, and baking sheet or grill, tongs

BAJA SLAW

1 cup cider vinegar

¼ cup honey

1 cup lime juice, room temp

1 small jalapeño, minced

⅔ bunch cilantro, minced

¼ head red cabbage, sliced

1 medium red or green pepper, julienned

1 large carrot, shredded

1. Whisk the cider vinegar and honey together in a medium-sized bowl, add the lime juice and whisk again.

2. Prep the vegetables. De-seed the jalapeño (or not for a spicier version). Mince and add to the bowl of marinade. Rinse, then de-stem the full bunch of cilantro. Mince ⅔ of the bunch and add to the bowl of marinade. Set aside the other third as a garnish for the completed tacos. Peel the outer 1-2 layers of the cabbage and cut out and discard the stem. Slice the cabbage to ⅛ - ¼-inch thick or use a mandolin. Add to the bowl of marinade and submerge. Julienne the pepper to ¼-inch. Add to the bowl. See Julienne Tip 27. Peel the carrot (or not) and shred it on a box grater. Add to the marinade and submerge.

3. Set a plate on the vegetables in the marinade and weigh it down with a can. Place in the fridge.

4. Marinate for at least two hours or up to two days before needed.

5. To serve, strain the veggies out of the marinade, place them in a serving bowl, and set aside. Toss, or keep the marinade for 1 week if you are going to make it again.

FISH TACO SEASONING

1 Tbsp granulated garlic

1 Tbsp iodized salt

1 Tbsp ground cumin

1 Tbsp dried ground mustard

1 ½ tsp chili powder

1 ½ tsp ground oregano

½ tsp cayenne

1. Combine all the spices in a small mixing bowl.

BUILDING THE TACOS

3-4 lbs whitefish (4 lbs w/skin, 3 lbs w/o skin)

1 Tbsp canola oil

2-3 whole avocados or 2 cups guacamole

½ pack 6-inch corn tortillas, g.f.

⅓ bunch cilantro

1. Heat the oven to broil or fire up the grill.

2. Cover a baking sheet with aluminum foil and a light layer of cooking oil. Lay out the fish so it is not overlapping. You may need two pans or to cook the fish in two batches.

3. Sprinkle each fish filet with approx. 1 teaspoon of Fish Taco Seasoning. If using an oven, bake for 6-10 minutes. If grilling, place foil and filets onto the grill. Note: Over-cooked fish is dry and rubbery, while perfectly cooked is steaming. Keep an eye on it.

4. Slice the avocados. See Avocado Tip 29. If using guacamole, skip this step.

5. Wrap the tortillas in slightly damp paper towels and microwave for 45 seconds. Set aside with a plate over them to retain warmth.

6. Set the cooked fish in your workspace. Gather the warm tortillas, strained Baja Slaw, avocado slices (or guacamole), and cilantro. To build tacos, lay out three tortillas and use tongs to divide 1 filet into each of the 3 tortillas. Add approx. ¼ cup Baja Slaw, and 2 slices of avocado per taco. Set on a plate, garnish with cilantro. Repeat.

recipe tip: Skin-on fish filets are preferable in this recipe. The cooked flesh will slide off the skin, leaving you with tender and moist fish. Without the skin, the fish can become crunchy or stick in the pan.

pro tip

Whitefish de-boning - If you feel a line of bones when sliding your fingers along the fish flesh, try this method. With a boning knife, (long, thin and flexible) cut close to each side of the line of bones, cutting down to the cutting board. Discard the boney strip. This is called the Channel method and is the quickest and easiest way to debone a whitefish.

I love that cafe. I stop every time I go through Duluth.
-Tony Bosak (line cook)

yucatan carnitas tacos

JILLIAN FORTE **2 HOURS 30 MINUTES** **SERVES 6 (3 TACOS EACH)** **DAIRY-FREE** **GLUTEN-FREE**

I have a serious soft spot for Mexican street tacos and try them in every state I explore south of the border. My favorite style is from the Yucatan, where the heat is sweltering and citrus grows in abundance. This recipe pays homage to the peninsula's carnitas, with simmering pork spiked with orange and lime juices. The result is a tender, bright, and versatile meat. The large recipe proportions here accommodate a Boston Butt or Picnic Shoulder cut (usually about 2-3 lbs). Any surplus meat can be portioned in zipper bags and frozen. Serve over rice, in enchiladas, quesadillas, or torta style in a hoagie bun.

gather

chef's knife, cutting board, heavy-bottomed rondeau & lid, measuring spoons, liquid measuring cups, wooden spoon

2-3 lbs pork butt

1 Tbsp canola oil

3+ cups water

2-4 tsp kosher salt, divided

2 tsp fresh minced garlic

2 bay leaves

1 yellow onion, minced, divided

½ bunch cilantro, minced

½ cup orange juice

2 Tbsp lime juice

2 tsp paprika

1 tsp dried oregano

1 Tbsp ground cumin

½ pack 6-inch corn tortillas, g.f.

1. Dice the pork to approx. 2-inches. If there is a bone, put it in the pot.

2. Pour the oil into a heavy-bottomed pot or rondeau. Add the meat, 2 teaspoons salt, garlic, bay leaves, and just enough water to cover the meat. Bring to a simmer over medium-high heat.

3. Cover and lower the heat. Let simmer for approx. 1.5 hours. Note: This can take up to 2 hours.

4. Check the meat for tenderness. The meat should flatten with the back of a wooden spoon. If not, continue to simmer, checking every 20 minutes.

5. While the meat is cooking, peel and finely mince the onion. Add half to the pot and recover. Reserve the remaining. De-stem and mince the cilantro. Mix with the reserved onion and place in a serving bowl.

6. Add the orange and lime juice, paprika, oregano, and cumin to the pork. Stir, cover, and simmer for 15 minutes.

7. Remove the lid and let the liquid start evaporating. Stir and break apart the meat as it simmers for 15-25 minutes, or until the liquid is almost gone.

8. Remove the bay leaves and any bones. Finish shredding the pork with a large spoon on the side of the pot or two forks. Taste the meat for salt and spice. See Salting Meat Tip.

9. Wrap the tortillas in slightly damp paper towels and microwave for 45 seconds.

10. Fill the tortillas with approx. ½ cup of carnitas meat. Serve with the cilantro-onion mix, hot sauce, salsa or Pico de Gallo 106, and fresh lime wedges. A salad of tomato and cucumber, lime juice, olive oil, salt, and pepper works great as a side!

recipe tip:

No two pieces of meat are ever the same size, so it's important to adjust spices and salt to find a balance for your taste buds. Always start with less salt. This recipe cooks out the water, so taste for salt after the water has evaporated. The same goes for the spice levels.

beef bulgogi tacos

JILLIAN FORTE **50 MINUTES** **SERVES 4-5**   **DAIRY-FREE**   **GLUTEN-FREE**

Korean bulgogi marinade tends toward sweet, so I modified this recipe to create a savory profile that I thought Cafe customers would enjoy. When preparing, resist the urge to skip the fish sauce. (I once spilled fish sauce on the floor beneath my workstation and all-day wondered where the rotten smell was coming from!) Despite its funky smell, fish sauce creates an umami flavor bomb that will raise your dish to a more complex level. This Beef Bulgogi is also great served with brown rice or rice noodles with a side of Massaged Kale Salad 136.

gather

chef knife and cutting board, mixing bowl, whisk, measuring spoons and cups, sauté pan or grill and grill tray

2 Tbsp white sugar

¾ tsp black pepper

¼ cup g.f. tamari, or soy sauce

1 Tbsp + 1 tsp sesame oil

1 Tbsp lime juice

1-2 tsp g.f. fish sauce

3 Tbsp minced green onion (approx. 1-2)

1 Tbsp +1 tsp fresh minced garlic

1 tsp fresh minced ginger

2 tsp canola oil

1-1½ lb beef

½ pack 6-inch corn tortillas or flour

1-2 cups Matt's Kimchi 109 or store-bought

1. Mix the sugar, black pepper, tamari, sesame oil, lime juice, and fish sauce in a medium-sized mixing bowl.

2. Mince the green onion, garlic, and ginger. Add to the bowl. Set aside.

3. Slice the beef against the grain, as thin as possible. Leave the meat as it collects on the side of the knife. When finished, turn the cutting board 45 degrees and cut the pile into 3-4-inch pieces.

4. Stir the meat into the marinade. Marinate for a minimum of ½ hour and up to 4 days. If marinating longer, be sure to label, date, and refrigerate covered.

5. Heat a sauté pan over medium-high heat and add the canola oil. Pour the meat and marinade into the pan. Cook for approximately 10-15 minutes, or until the marinade covers the meat in a glossy dark, flavorful sauce. Note: This will be longer than you think. There shouldn't be liquid left in the pan. If there is, keep cooking until it has evaporated. Alternatively, you can grill the meat. Use a grill tray so the thin slices don't fall through the cracks.

6. Wrap the tortillas in slightly damp paper towels and microwave for 45 seconds.

7. Pile bowls with the Bulgogi beef, kimchi, and tortillas. Build your own tacos and dig in!

pro tip

Partially frozen meat is easier to thinly slice.

vegan bulgogi tacos

JILLIAN FORTE **50 MINUTES** **SERVES 4-5**   **GLUTEN-FREE**   **VEGAN**   **DAIRY-FREE**

The vegan version of our Bulgogi Tacos is made with tempeh and mushrooms, but you can substitute tofu for tempeh, or combine mushrooms and onion. This marinade gets its umami from the miso and is as versatile as vegans are creative!

gather

chef knife and cutting board, mixing bowl, whisk, measuring spoons and cups, sauté pan

2 Tbsp white sugar

¾ tsp black pepper

¼ cup + g.f. tamari or soy sauce

1 Tbsp + 1 tsp sesame oil

1 Tbsp lime juice

1-2 tsp miso, brown or red

3 Tbsp minced green onion (approx. 1-2)

1 Tbsp +1 tsp fresh minced garlic

1 tsp fresh minced ginger

2 tsp canola oil

1 lb mushrooms (shiitake, chicken of the woods, or oysters)

8 oz tempeh

½ pack 6-inch corn tortilla or flour

1 cup Matt's Kimchi 109 or store-bought

1. Mix the sugar, black pepper, tamari, sesame oil, lime juice, and miso into a medium-sized mixing bowl.

2. Mince the green onion, garlic, and ginger. Add to the bowl. Stir together and taste. You can add a bit more tamari to balance out the sweetness in the miso.

3. Dice the tempeh into ½-inch cubes and mix with the marinade.

4. Slice the mushrooms to about ¼-inch, then in half once (if using shiitakes, de-stem). Add to the bowl and mix. Marinate for 15 minutes and up to 24 hours.

5. Heat a sauté pan over medium-high heat and add the canola oil. Wait one minute and add the tempeh/mushroom mix, and all the juices. The marinade will cook down, covering the tempeh and mushrooms in a glossy dark, flavorful sauce.

6. Wrap the tortillas in slightly damp paper towels and microwave for 45 seconds.

7. Pile bowls with the Bulgogi mushrooms and tempeh, kimchi, and tortillas. Build your own tacos and dig in!

Carla once hired St. Olaf's Choir to perform at St. Scholastica. The following morning, they all ate breakfast at the restaurant. When finished, they sang an acapella song that filled the restaurant. "It was just one of those memorable jobs."
- Collen Betts (night chef)

Lynda and I were regulars at Chester Creek Cafe At Sara's Table for many years prior to moving to Bozeman, MT. The Cafe not only provided delicious food, but had great servers, chefs, and other staff. We befriended several staff members over the years. Many were in our social network of friends prior to moving to MT. We were invited to cafe gatherings as well and had several parties over at our place. A former server and her son visited us while in Bozeman last summer. While in Duluth this June, we were having breakfast At Sara's Table, and in walked 5 former servers for a reunion. So great to see all of them. Also, Lynda was part of the Diners, Drive-Ins, and Dives when Guy taped a segment for his show at the restaurant. This Cafe has become, and will always be, a special place for us and for anyone who dines there.
- Lee Dietrich (customer & friend)

Recent nicknames for the ladies are Barla and Carbon or Carbar and Barcla! Obviously born from trying to say their names too fast.

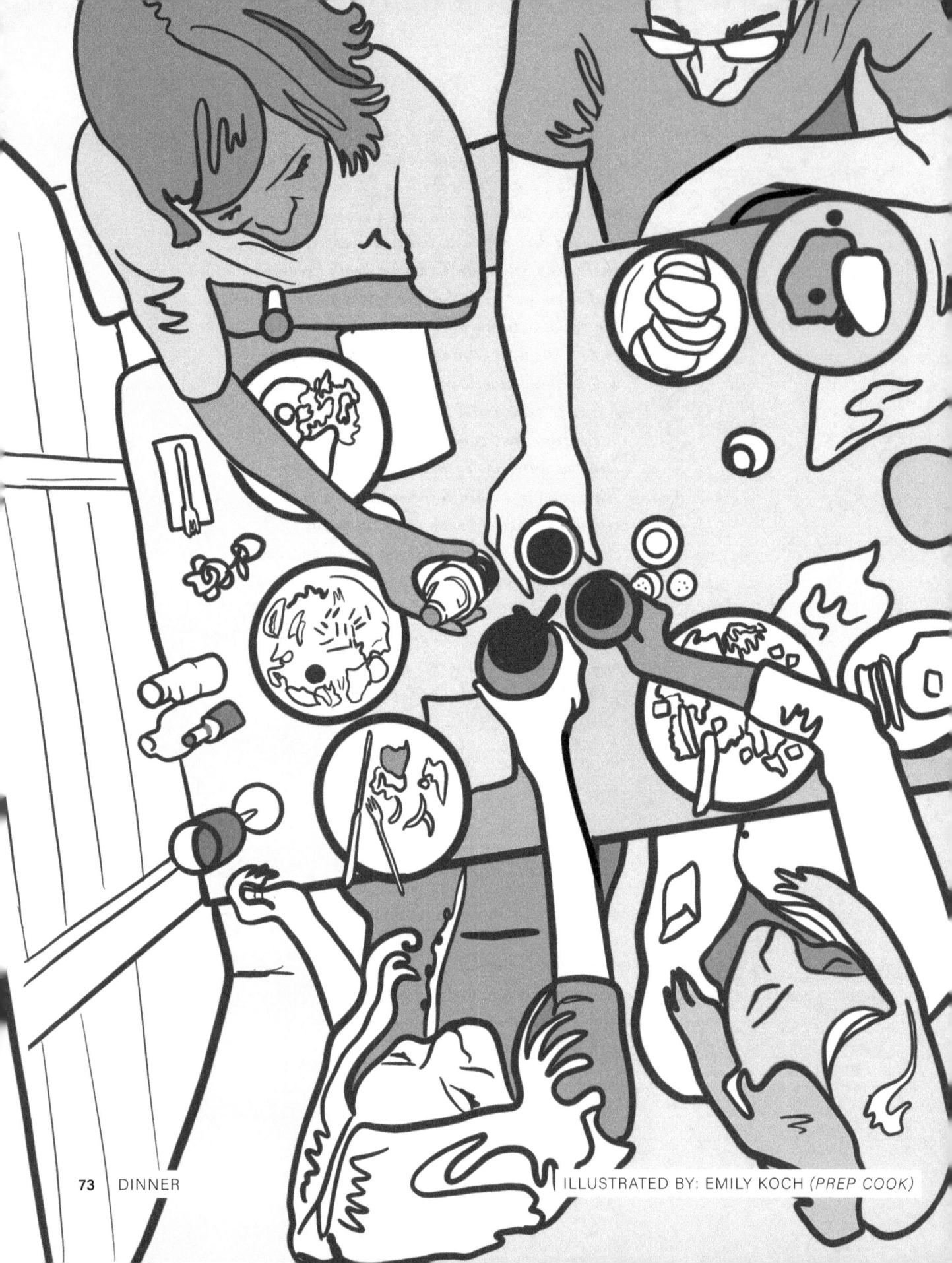

ILLUSTRATED BY: EMILY KOCH (*PREP COOK*)

dinner

After a busy day at the Cafe, the mood at dinner shifts palpably. People are no longer rushing off to accomplish their daily tasks, but rather decompressing over the final meal of the day. The calming energy of evening invites the urge to lounge and linger. In the depth of Minnesota winters, when the sun sets in the afternoon, customers dine in cozy comfort, happy to have fought off the tendency to hibernate. In the summer, when the patio is blanketed in warmth, and the day stretches into a seductive blue evening, the relaxed atmosphere begs for dessert, or perhaps an extra glass of wine. Dinner allows time to savor more complex flavor profiles. You'll find them reflected in the Cafes' eclectic dinner menu.

Unique to this section of the cookbook, most dinner recipes offer a complete meal, including sides, and "timing instructions" for efficient preparation. Still, you can easily make one element of the recipe. If you prefer to mix and match, browse the Small Plates, Sauces & Bonuses section for more options. Some recipes allow for prepping ahead, while others are portioned to create extras, perfect for freezing and reheating in a pinch. Quite a few of the dinners here are "date night" worthy. Prepare them with a date, or for a date, and enjoy a glamorous evening together.

cabernet braised beef & crispy polenta

NATALIE ALLESEE **7-8 HOURS** **SERVES 8** **GLUTEN-FREE**

Braising a chuck roast low and slow lends a gloriously tender texture to a piece of meat known for fat and rich texture. The addition of copious amounts of red wine, aromatics, tomato, and mushroom make this dish luxurious and decadent. The braising and shredding of the beef creates a Bolognese-style meal. It is also excellent served over homemade gnocchi or pasta. For a romantic night in, enjoy this dish in candlelight along with a fat glass of your favorite Bordeaux, or make it the center of a glamorous dinner party, and share!

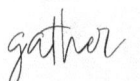 **Dutch oven, rondeau or heavy-bottomed 8-quart stockpot, chef knife, cutting board, tongs, cheesecloth, measuring cups and spoons, blender, sauce pot, whisk, spatula, glass pie pan or 6 x 6 pan, sauté pan**

BRAISED BEEF

2 cups red peppers, chopped (approx. 2)

2 cups yellow onion, quartered (approx. 1)

2 Tbsp fresh minced garlic

1 ¾ cups Cabernet Sauvignon or any boxed red wine

2 lb chuck roast

5 Tbsp canola oil

2 tsp kosher salt

2 Tbsp black peppercorns

3 bay leaves

1 ¾ cups beef stock

2- 14.5oz cans diced tomatoes

1. De-seed and rough chop the red peppers. See Pepper Tip 28. Peel and quarter the yellow onion. Mince 2 tablespoons of garlic.

2. Trim the chuck roast as much as you like or not at all. Fat adds richness. The buried sinew will become soft and easy to remove when you shred the beef in the final steps.

3. Heat the dutch oven over medium-high heat until hot and add the oil. While the pot is heating, cover the beef with the salt. Sear the roast on all sides, using tongs to turn as needed. Set the beef aside.

4. Sauté the red peppers and onions for 4-5 minutes. Add the garlic. Cook for an additional minute. Add the wine and beef.

5. Place the peppercorns and bay leaves into a piece of cheesecloth. Roll and tie the ends. Place inside the pot with the beef.

6. Reduce the heat to medium. Simmer until the wine is reduced in half.

7. Add the beef stock and tomatoes to the pot. Stir, cover, and lower the heat. Let simmer, slightly bubbling, for 3-4 hours. Check occasionally to make sure the liquid hasn't evaporated from an ill-fitting lid. If it has, add more beef stock or water.

   🔔 Start the polenta now.

8. The meat is done when it is "fall-apart tender". At the Cafe, we often let the beef cool overnight in the liquid. Like a soup, the flavors will intensify with time. However, you can move directly to the next step.

9. Remove the cheesecloth sachet and discard. Set the beef into a bowl to cool. Pour the liquid and vegetables into a blender and puree until very fine, set aside.

CRISPY POLENTA

5 cups water

2 cups half & half

1 ½ tsp kosher salt

2 cup polenta aka corn meal

4 Tbsp salted butter

2 Tbsp heavy cream

¾ cup shredded Parmesan

½ tsp black pepper

1 Tbsp canola oil

1. Boil the water and half & half in a medium-sized sauce pot. Add salt and reduce heat to medium-low.

2. Pour the polenta into the water in a steady stream, while whisking. Continue whisking until free of clumps.

3. Cook and whisk or stir frequently until the polenta pulls away from the sides of the pot. Test a small bit to ensure it is thoroughly soft. Note: The thickness of the grind of the cornmeal will determine the length of the cooking time. A finely ground cornmeal will cook for 5 minutes while a coarser grind can take up to 40 minutes.

4. Add the butter, heavy cream, Parmesan, and black pepper. Stir until the cheese has melted.

5. Pour the creamy polenta into a round or square baking pan. Use a clean wet rubber spatula to spread it around until an even thickness. Place in the fridge uncovered until chilled, approx 2 hours.

🔔 If making the whole dish, make the Cabernet Sauce while waiting.

6. Use a spatula to loosen the edges of the chilled polenta from the pan. Place a cutting board on top of the dish and flip both over, remove the baking pan. The polenta will suction itself out. Cut the polenta into 8 even-sized pieces.

7. Heat a sauté pan over medium-high heat. Add the canola oil and wait until the oil runs quickly over the pan indicating that the pan is hot enough. Place as many pieces of polenta into the pan as will fit with space around them. Sear until golden and crispy. Flip and sear the other side. Repeat until all pieces are seared.

CABERNET SAUCE

3 ½ cups yellow onion, minced (approx. 2)

2 Tbsp fresh minced garlic

5 cups shiitake mushroom caps, sliced (approx. 2- 5oz containers)

½ cup canola oil

1 Tbsp kosher salt

2 Tbsp fresh minced thyme

2 Tbsp fresh minced oregano

1 ¾ cups Cabernet Sauvignon or red wine

1. Mince the yellow onions. Mince the garlic. De-stem the shiitake mushrooms (discard the stems or reserve them for stock). Slice the caps to ¼ -inch and set aside. De-stem and mince the thyme and oregano.

2. Heat a heavy-bottomed 8-quart pot or large rondeau over medium heat, add the oil and wait one minute. Sauté the onions until translucent, 3-4 minutes.

3. Add and cook the mushrooms until soft, 3-4 minutes. Add the garlic and salt, and cook for one minute.

4. Add the herbs and wine. Boil, uncovered until the liquid reduces by half.

5. While the wine is reducing, hand shred the meat. Remove large clumps of fat or sinew.

🔔 If making the whole dish, start searing the polenta after the meat is shredded.

6. Once the wine has reduced, pour in the blended veggies from the braising and add the shredded beef. Stir and taste for salt. Pour over the crispy polenta and garnish with extra minced herbs.

grilled jerk chicken
& coconut cauliflower "rice"

JILLIAN FORTE **1 DAY + 40 MINUTES** **SERVES 4** **GLUTEN-FREE** **KETO** **DAIRY-FREE**

This Keto-friendly dish is a fun and flavor-forward take on grilled chicken. Traditionally, Jerk Chicken is cooked over smoldering green Pimento logs, which lends the meat a pungent flavor. Since Pimento trees don't grow in Minnesota, this recipe uses allspice berries and bay leaves to imbue the meat with a subtle earthy flavor. Admittedly, the accompanying cauliflower "rice" sounds like a food fad. Let me assure you it's not only delicious, and easy to make, but it's a great way to reduce carbs while adding more vegetables to your diet. Pre-riced cauliflower is available at most grocery stores, however, a food processor makes it quick to do at home.

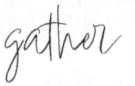

chef knife, cutting board, paring knife, disposable gloves, citrus juicer, zester, small and medium-sized mixing bowls, measuring spoons, rubber spatula, plastic wrap or gallon zipper bags, small sealable container, medium-sized saucepot, grill, tongs

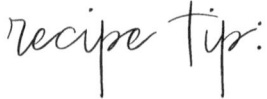

Habanero and Scotch Bonnet peppers are extremely spicy. It's best to wear disposable gloves, and to wash the knife, cutting board, and hands directly after working with them. If you cut the peppers with bare hands, try using dish soap to cut the burn.

COCONUT CAULIFLOWER "RICE"

1 Tbsp coconut oil

1 cup red pepper, ¼-inch dice (approx. 1 small)

4 cups riced cauliflower (approx. 1 medium)

1 ½ tsp kosher salt

1- 5.4 oz can coconut milk

¼ cup water

1 Tbsp lime juice

1 Tbsp fresh minced cilantro

1. Dice the red pepper to ¼-inch. De-stem and mince the cilantro. To make cauliflower rice, rough chop the cauliflower. Half-fill your food processor (or quarter-fill a blender). Run the machine until the pieces are rice-sized. Continue in batches until you've made 4 cups.

2. Heat the saucepot over medium heat, add the coconut oil, and wait one minute.

3. Add and sauté the red peppers until soft, about 3 minutes.

4. Add the cauliflower and salt. Cook and stir until the cauliflower begins to brown, about 10 minutes. If the cauliflower scorches, dribble in a little water and stir. You want the cauliflower to be soft but not sloppy wet.

5. Add the coconut milk. This will form steam and help the cooking process.

   🔔 Fire up your grill for the chicken.

6. Cook and stir for 10-15 minutes, then turn off the heat. Stir in 1 tablespoon of reserved lime juice and minced cilantro.

7. Taste the cauliflower and add more salt or lime juice to your preference. There is a balance between acid and salt that is perfect, though different, for each person's palate. Experiment until you find it!

JERK CHICKEN

1 Tbsp minced Habanero or Scotch Bonnet pepper (approx. 1)

2 Tbsp minced green onion (approx. 1-2)

2 tsp fresh minced ginger

2 tsp fresh minced garlic

2 tsp fresh minced thyme

1 tsp ground allspice

½ tsp ground nutmeg

1 tsp kosher salt

½ tsp black pepper

2 Tbsp g.f. tamari, or soy sauce

1 Tbsp canola oil

2 tsp lime zest (approx. 1 large lime)

1 Tbsp lime juice

1 whole chicken or pre-quartered

2 Tbsp whole allspice berries

12-16 bay leaves

1. De-seed and mince the Habanero pepper. Warning, wear gloves! Place into a medium-sized mixing bowl. Wash hands, cutting board, and knife.

2. Mince the green onion, ginger, garlic, and fresh thyme. Add to the bowl.

3. Add the ground allspice, nutmeg, salt, pepper, tamari, and oil to the bowl.

4. Fully zest one lime, measuring the zest is unnecessary. Forcefully roll the lime on the table under the palm of your hand to break the capillaries. Juice the lime into a small bowl. Add 1 tablespoon of the juice to the bowl of spices, and reserve the remaining juice for the Coconut Cauliflower Rice. Mix the marinade.

5. If using a whole chicken, cut it into quarters (reserve the backbone for stock). If "breaking down" a chicken is new to you, watching a video will be very helpful as it's difficult to explain without hands-on instruction.

6. Score the chicken by slicing a cross-hatch into the skin of the chicken. Occasionally cut through the skin, allowing the marinade to penetrate the flesh. Note: If you use skinless chicken, there is no need to score the meat.

7. Place the chicken pieces into the bowl of marinade. Use a rubber spatula to coat each piece.

8. Cover the mixing bowl with plastic wrap. Or place the chicken and marinade into a large zip top plastic bag. Push all the air out of the bag and seal. Marinate for 4 hours and up to 2 days.

9. In a sealable container, cover the allspice berries and bay leaves in water. Store in the fridge next to or on top of the marinating chicken. You don't want to forget this ingredient!

FINALE

1. Push the soaked allspice berries and bay leaves into the bottom side of the chicken. Put on a slotted grill tray, if you have one, or directly onto the grill. When the spices fall into the flames, the resulting smoke will impart flavor to the chicken.

2. Cook the chicken, rotating as necessary until it is done. Pull off any bay leaves or allspice berries before serving.

3. Divide the Coconut Cauliflower Rice onto four plates and add a chicken piece to each. This meal is ready to serve!

lamb kefta kabobs, tzatziki & fresh pita bread

**JILLIAN FORTE &
RITA B. BERGSTEDT**

 1 HOUR, 20 MINUTES   **4 (TWO KABOBS & 1 PITA EACH)**   *GLUTEN-FREE   *KETO

Every season when evaluating menus, I often grouped sales according to protein choice: chicken, beef, vegetarian, and so on, but there were always menu items that were 'other.' I lovingly refer to those who order 'other' dishes as the adventurous diners. Creating dishes for them adds spice to a chef's life! This Kefta Kabob recipe (you'll find many versions of kabob from Turkey to Morocco) exemplifies an adventurous dish. Made with lamb, it introduces the flavors of both sumac and Urfa pepper. Add creamy Tzatziki and surprisingly easy-to-make Fresh Pita Bread, and the entire dish can be served in either a wrap or as a plated dinner.

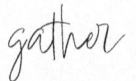 liquid measuring cup, measuring spoons, fork, plastic wrap, chef knife, cutting board, peeler, spoon, box grater, plate, fine-mesh strainer, 2-3 mixing bowls, skewers, rolling pin, grill, tongs or metal spatula

TZATZIKI SAUCE

1 cucumber, peeled and shredded

3 Tbsp red onion, minced (approx. ¼)

½ tsp fresh minced garlic

1 cup plain Greek yogurt (Greek Gods)

¾ tsp dried dill

1 ½ tsp lemon juice

1 Tbsp + 1 ½ tsp extra virgin olive oil

¼ tsp kosher salt

⅛ tsp black pepper

🔔   If making the whole dish, start with the Fresh Pita Bread.

1. Peel and remove the ends from the cucumber. Slice it down the middle lengthwise. Scrape out the seeds with a spoon, and discard. Halve the cucumber length-wise.

2. Place the grater on a plate and shred the cucumber (using two quarters at a time works well). Put the grated cucumber in a fine-mesh strainer and push out the excess liquid. Discard (or drink) the juice and place the grated cucumber in a mixing bowl.

3. Mince and measure out the red onion and garlic. Add to the mixing bowl.

4. Add the yogurt, dill, lemon juice, olive oil, salt, and pepper. Mix and taste. Chill until serving time.

FRESH PITA BREAD

RITA B. BERGSTEDT

¾ cup warm water

1 tsp active dry yeast

½ tsp white sugar

1 ¾ + cups all-purpose flour

⅓ cup whole wheat flour

1 tsp kosher salt

1+ Tbsp extra virgin olive oil

1. Put ¾ cup of warm water in a liquid measuring cup. Add the active yeast and sugar. Stir until dissolved. Let it rest until it foams up, approx. 5 minutes.

2. Put the flours in a mixing bowl. Add the salt and mix.

3. Pour the foamy water-yeast mixture and 1 tablespoon of olive oil into the flour. Mix with either a fork or in the bowl of a stand mixer using the dough hook until evenly combined.

4. If you have a stand mixer, knead the dough in the bowl. Otherwise, turn the dough out onto a floured work surface and knead for approx. 4-5 minutes. Roll the dough into a ball. Stretch the dough so there is a single seam on the bottom of the dough. See the Pro Tip on stretching dough.

5. Coat the inside of a clean mixing bowl with a little olive oil. Place the dough ball in the bowl and roll it around until it is coated in oil. Leave it seam side down in the bowl and cover with plastic wrap. Place in a warm spot and let rise until it has doubled in size, about one hour.

   🔔 If making the whole dish, move on to the Tzatziki and Kebobs.

6. Remove the pita dough onto a floured surface and flatten it to remove the air bubbles. Cut the dough into 4-5 equal pieces. Do not knead the dough but pull the edges to a single point to form a tight ballon. Set it aside with the seam on the bottom. Let it rest for 10-15 minutes.

   🔔 If making the whole dish, fire up the grill before this step. Put Kabobs on the grill while the dough is resting.

7. Using a rolling pin, roll each dough ball into a 4-6-inch wide circle. Grill or place in an oiled sauté pan over medium heat. You can cook only one pita at a time in a pan, whereas a grill has room for many. Cook on each side until browned, or a little singed.

   🔔 If plating up the entire dish, move to the Finale.

---

pro Tip

Stretching dough - Lay dough on a floured work surface. Fold the dough in thirds, flatten, rotate 90 degrees, and fold in thirds again. Pick up the dough ball and turn it over so the folds are towards the table. Now gently pull the sides of the dough down to the bottom until the dough looks like a tight balloon. Turn the dough over and pinch and twist the seams together. Place the dough ball seam down to let the dough rest.

KEFTA KABOBS

1 medium yellow onion, shredded *sub ½ cup minced green onion

2 Tbsp fresh minced parsley

1 Tbsp fresh minced mint

1 lb ground lamb

2 tsp domestic paprika

1 ½ tsp ground cumin

1 ½ tsp Urfa pepper or sweet smoked paprika or Aleppo peppers

1 ½ tsp sumac or 1 tsp lemon zest

¾ tsp kosher salt

¼ tsp black pepper

🔔 If using wooden skewers, soak them in water now.

1. Cut the stem, not the root side, off of the onion. Peel back the onion skin and leave it hanging off the root end.

2. Shred the onions on a box grate by holding onto the stem and skin. Grating will create a large amount of liquid, so set the grater on a plate. Put the grated onion into a fine-mesh strainer and push out as much of the liquid as possible. Place the onion pulp into a mixing bowl and discard the liquid.

3. Mince the parsley and mint. Add to the bowl.

4. Add the ground lamb and the dry spices. Mix well with your hands.

5. Divide the meat into 8 even-sized portions. Shape each portion, compacting it as much as possible, into a flattened oval, about 3-inches long by 2-inches wide. Skewer through the long way, one portion per skewer.

6. Fire up the grill. You can also use a sauté pan, in which case don't fire up the grill!

🔔 If making the whole dish, return to Fresh Pita Bread, step 6.

7. Cook the kabobs in either a sauté pan or on the grill until done. Note: This meat can be crumbly as there is no binder. If you are grilling, use a slotted grill tray.

FINALE

ENTRÉE OR WRAP

1. For a plated entrée, cut each pita into 4-6 triangles, and fan out on a plate with tips pointing outwards. Place 2 skewered kabobs and a side dish of tzatziki on each plate.

2. For a wrap, take four squares of aluminum foil and fold each one opposite corner to corner into a triangle. Place the pita on top of the foil. Put the un-skewered kabobs inside the pita and pour tzatziki over the top. Fold the pita in half and wrap it in the foil.

Barb and Carla are wonderful. They have giant hearts. Their priority is not to make money, but to make sure their people are taken care of. We are kind of like this tribe of adult children who follow them around. I have been admonished more than once, and I have been celebrated more than once. For instance, Barb said I made the best Mojitos she's ever had, and to get my damn skirt longer. She was always real. Barb and Carla care about the neighborhood and the community. They are unapologetic and vocal about social issues which made me really, really proud to work there. - Melissa Weisser (server)

Al Franken came to the Cafe years ago while running for office. I was a fan of his radio show before he was on SNL, so I wormed my way up to see him. I asked if he'd like a tour of the restaurant and he agreed! That's how I got my picture taken with him. - Diane Bailey (baker)

green buddha bowl & tahini sauce

HEATHER ERICKSON **55 MINUTES** **SERVES 2**   **GLUTEN-FREE**   **VEGAN**   **DAIRY-FREE**

Heather, the creator of yet another Cafe favorite, defines the Buddha Bowl as "a healthy, protein-packed, plant-based meal." Its whole grain base supports a flavorful sauce and piles of sautéed vegetables, vegetarian proteins, seeds, or nuts, and often avocado as a healthy fat. The resulting dish delights in taste, texture, and color. Add your own favorite toppings. I love my Buddha Bowl with kimchi and a tamari egg!

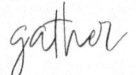 **2 medium pots, 2 mixing bowls, blender, chef knife, cutting board, strainer, measuring cups and spoons, 2 sauté pans**

GREEN BUDDHA BOWL

2 ½ cups water

1 cup brown rice,
long or medium grain

2 cups broccoli florets
(approx. half a small head)

½ tray ice cubes

**2 cups Kale Salad 136, or
8 leaves of raw kale**

6 oz tempeh

**1 Tbsp T&T Marinade 121,
or g.f. tamari**

2 tsp sesame seeds,
toasted

4 Tbsp pepitas, toasted

2 Tbsp canola oil, divided

1 cup shelled edamame

1 tsp mirin

2 tsp fresh minced garlic

**2 tsp fresh minced
ginger**

**2-4 Tbsp Tahini Sauce,
recipe follows**

½ tsp kosher salt

1 avocado

1. Boil 2 ½ cups of water in a medium-sized pot. Add the rice, cover, and gently simmer until cooked, approx. 30 minutes.

2. Boil 2-3 quarts of water in a medium pot. Cut the broccoli into bite-sized florets and set aside.

3. Prepare the Kale Salad 136. If choosing raw kale, which is quicker and simpler, de-stem and cut the kale into approx. 2-inch squares. See Kale Tip 29.

4. Put half a tray of ice and cold water into a medium-sized bowl. Plunge the broccoli into the boiling water, and wait 1 minute, or until it turns a bright green. Strain, then quickly submerge into the ice water. Once the broccoli is chilled, strain it again and let it drip dry in the sink until needed.

5. Cut the tempeh into ½-inch squares. Put into a small bowl and pour either T&T Marinade 121 or tamari over it. Toss gently to coat, and set aside.

6. Cut the avocado in half and remove the pit. Slice the avocado while in the skin and set aside. See Avocado Tip 29.

   🔔 If making the Tahini Sauce, do so now.

7. Heat a sauté pan over medium heat. Add the sesame seeds and pepitas. Stir and toast for approx. 3 minutes or until lightly brown. Set aside to cool.

8. Add 1 tablespoon canola oil, the blanched broccoli, and edamame to the hot sauté pan. Sauté for 3-4 minutes or until the edamame blisters.

9. Add the garlic, ginger, and salt to the pan. If using raw kale, add it now. Cook for 1 minute.

10. Deglaze the pan with the mirin. Turn off the heat. Set aside in the pan to keep it warm. If you only have one sauté pan, pour the vegetables into a bowl and cover.

11. Put a sauté pan on medium-high heat and add the remaining tablespoon of canola oil. Remove the tempeh from the marinade and put it into the sauté pan, watch out for splashing oil. Sauté until browned, about 5 minutes.

12. Divide the cooked rice into two wide bowls. Pour 1-2 tablespoons of Tahini Sauce on each pile of rice. Arrange the prepared ingredients: broccoli & edamame, kale salad, avocado, and tempeh on top of the rice. Sprinkle with sesame seeds and pepitas. Serve with tamari and your favorite hot sauce.

TAHINI SAUCE

2 Tbsp water

2 Tbsp g.f. tamari

2 Tbsp lime juice

1 Tbsp tahini or peanut butter

¼ tsp kosher salt

½ tsp Sriracha

1. Blend all the ingredients together in a food processor or blender.

---

pro tip

Avoid stirring rice, unless it's risotto. Stirring will agitate the starches and leave the rice sticky and clumpy. After you have turned off the heat, fluff the rice just enough to get the rice from the bottom to the top. Return the cover and let the residual heat steam any slightly underdone kernels.

I worked for two queer women at the forefront of the environmental scene. I slept soundly at night because I worked for a company that believed in social justice issues, was environmentally conscious, and supported the local community. It was nice working with like-minded people. I made lifelong friendships there. I was well-trusted, so I felt appreciated.
- Jon Choi (FoH manager)

vietnamese braised beef short ribs & garlic chili sauce

CARLA BLUMBERG   **3 HOURS, 30 MINUTES** **SERVES 4** **GLUTEN-FREE** **DAIRY-FREE**

This incredibly rich and delicious dish has graced our menu many times throughout the years. Here it is served with rice noodles, Garlic Chili Sauce, and all the fixings. I like to add Kung Fu slaw 63 or Massaged Kale Salad 136. The skill it takes to brown the ribs perfectly on all sides will likely become a point of pride and satisfaction. Remember to taste test as you go. There will be leftover crunchy bits on the bottom of the pan!

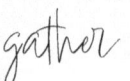 **gather**   chef knife and cutting board, rondeau or heavy-bottomed pot, measuring spoons, liquid measuring cup, tongs, medium bowl, roasting pan with lid or aluminum foil, small heavy-bottomed saucepot, mixing spoon, medium pot, strainer

RIBS

½ medium red onion, chopped

1 inch ginger, sliced

2 lbs beef short ribs, boneless ribs, or a combination

1-2 Tbsp kosher salt

1 Tbsp black pepper

2 Tbsp sesame oil

2 Tbsp canola oil

1 ½ cups mirin

1- 13.5 oz can full-fat coconut milk (Chaokoh)

2 cups beef stock

½ cup g.f. tamari or soy sauce

1 lime, wedged

2 green onions, thinly sliced

4 twigs fresh mint, de-stemmed

½ - 1 cup roaasted peanuts

1- 14 oz pack rice noodles, straight cut, thick

1. Heat the oven to 350°. Rough chop the red onions and thinly slice the ginger. Set both aside.

2. Cut the ribs into individual pieces; one bone per piece. Rinse the ribs in cold water, while gently rubbing the sides, then let them drip dry or dab with a paper towel. If boneless beef, cut into 2-inch cubes. FYI: Ribs are cut with a heavy-duty saw, which leaves bone fragments peppering the meat. It is important to remove them with a rinse.

3. Sprinkle the ribs (and/or cubed meat) with the salt and pepper.

4. Heat a heavy-bottomed rondeau over medium-high heat, then add the sesame and canola oils. When hot, place the ribs in the pan so they are not touching - overcrowding isn't good for seared meat. Sear each side until dark brown, using tongs to flip the meat as necessary. Put the seared pieces into a bowl to collect any juices. See Pro Tip 152.

5. Deglaze the empty pan with mirin. Be careful as the steam or splatter can burn.

6. Add the coconut milk, beef stock, and tamari. Mix until the coconut milk fats have dissolved.

7. Place the beef in a single layer on the bottom of the rondeau. Scatter in the red onions and the ginger. If the liquid does not completely cover the beef, use a smaller pan, or add a little more beef stock, mirin and tamari to top it off.

8. Cover the pan with aluminum foil and tightly seal. If it splits open, place the lid on the pan as well. Braise in the oven for 3 hours.

   🔔 If making the whole dish, set a timer for 2 ½ hours. Reset the timer for 30 minutes and start the Chili Garlic Sauce, then the Finale instructions.

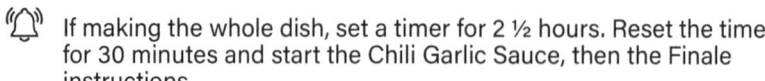 *recipe tip:* Short ribs vary in size and the ratio of meat to bone. Buy two ribs per person. If the ribs are not very meaty, or you can't find bone-in, substitute boneless short ribs and cut the beef into 2 x 2-inch pieces.

GARLIC CHILI SAUCE

2 Tbsp fresh minced ginger

1 Tbsp fresh minced garlic

½ tsp red pepper flakes

½ cup rice vinegar

1 Tbsp sesame oil

1 Tbsp Sriracha

2 Tbsp mirin

¼ cup white sugar

1. Peel and mince the garlic and ginger into tiny pieces.

2. Put the ginger, garlic, red pepper flakes, vinegar, oil, Sriracha, and mirin in a small heavy-bottomed saucepan. Bring to a boil, then lower heat to medium and simmer for 5 minutes.

3. Add the sugar, stir, and reduce the heat to medium-low. Simmer until thickened, 5-10 minutes. Allow the sauce to cool in the pan. The final product should be syrupy.

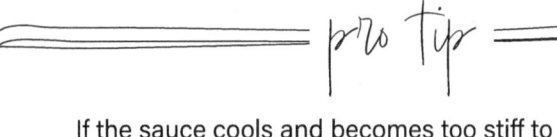

pro tip

If the sauce cools and becomes too stiff to pour, place the pan on low heat and stir in small amounts of warm water until the sauce returns to the proper consistency. I have seen this recipe over-cooked to the point a spoon could stand up in the pot. The sauce can be rescued!

FINALE

1. Set a pot of 2-3 quarts of water on to boil (2 ½ hours after the ribs have gone in the oven). Cut the lime into wedges, thinly slice the green onions, and de-stem the mint. Place these garnishes on a plate and set aside.

2. Follow the directions on the package of the rice noodles or see Rice Noodle Tip 29. Once the noodles are soft but not falling apart, strain and run lukewarm water over them. You want to stop the cooking process but keep them warm enough to eat. Drizzle a little sesame oil over the noodles.

3. Pull the ribs out of the oven and test for tenderness. When the meat is almost falling off the bone, gently pull them out of the liquid with the tongs.

4. Divide the rice noodles onto each plate and top with two ribs per plate. Garnish with lime wedges, green onions, mint, roasted peanuts, and a dish of Chili Garlic Sauce.

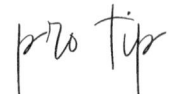

pro tip

Keep the leftover rib braising liquid. You can reduce it and use it as a sauce. Or add beef stock and used it as a soup base with rice noodles.

moroccan chicken tagine & couscous

JILLIAN FORTE   **1 HOUR & 30 MINUTES**   **SERVES 5-6** ***GLUTEN-FREE**

It's the warm deep spice mix Ras el Hanout, paired with classic stew ingredients, that makes this a winner on cold winter evenings. The recipe's fun additions of preserved lemons, olives, and apricots make it oh so memorable! (Ras el Hanout, and preserved lemons, can often be found in a grocery store's ethnic section, though sometimes the lemons are shelved near the pickles.) At the Cafe, we brine the chicken first (an easy step that yields a juicy and more flavorful bird), but skip brining if you're short on time. Serve over brown rice for a gluten-free version. Remember, one-pot meals are a blessing, especially to the dishwasher!

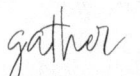 medium to large pot, dutch oven or rondeau, chef knife, cutting board, tongs, medium bowl, measuring cups and spoons, slotted spoon

DRY BRINE THE CHICKEN (optional)

1 whole chicken, or pre-cut bone-in

2-4 Tbsp kosher salt (optional)

1. Coat the chicken in kosher salt. Note: This may seem like a lot of salt, but you will rinse it off. Place in the fridge uncovered for 12-48 hours.

RAS EL HANOUT

1 Tbsp sweet or domestic paprika

2 tsp turmeric

1 ½ tsp smoked paprika

1 ½ tsp ground cumin

1 ½ tsp ginger powder

1 tsp ground allspice

1 tsp cayenne

1 tsp iodized salt

1 tsp ground cinnamon

¾ tsp ground cardamom

¼ tsp garlic powder

¼ tsp black pepper

1. Combine all the ingredients in a small mixing bowl.

COUSCOUS

3 cups vegetable stock or water

1 tsp salt

1 ½ cups couscous

2 Tbsp extra virgin olive oil

1. Bring the vegetable stock or water to a boil. Add the salt and couscous. Cover and remove from the heat.

2. When the timer for the Tagine goes off, fluff the couscous with a fork. Drizzle the extra virgin olive oil over the couscous and combine.

TAGINE

2 cups diced parsnips, 1-inch (approx. 2 parsnips)

2 cups diced Yukon gold potatoes, 1-inch (approx. 3)

2 cups diced yellow onions, ½-inch (approx. 1 large)

2 Tbsp fresh minced garlic

1 Tbsp + 1 ½ tsp fresh minced ginger

½ tray ice cubes

2 medium tomatoes

1 ½ tsp kosher salt

2 Tbsp canola oil

2 Tbsp tomato paste

4 cups chicken stock

1 pinch saffron

3 Tbsp minced preserved lemon or 2 fresh lemons juiced + salt

1 ½ cups pitted Castelvetrano olives or green olives

¾ cup dried apricots, quartered

2 Tbsp olive juice

1. Put 1-2 quarts of water on high heat to boil.

2. Rinse the salt from the chicken. If you are using a whole chicken, cut it into 8 pieces. If you are new to "breaking down" a chicken, a video will be very helpful. Remember to sanitize any surface the raw chicken touches.

3. Sprinkle the chicken pieces with 2+ tablespoons of Ras el Hanout.

4. Fill a mixing bowl with ½ tray of ice cubes and cold water. Take each of the tomatoes and score once, just through the skin. Place them in the boiling water with tongs. As soon as the skin peels, pull them out of the water and submerge them in the ice bath. Let cool for approx. 1 minute. Peel the tomatoes, discard the skins, cut in quarters or 8ths from stem to tip, and de-seed.

5. Peel, then dice the onions to approx. ½-inch - set aside in a bowl. Peel and mince the garlic and ginger. Place together in a small bowl. Peel, then dice the parsnips to 1-inch. Dice the potatoes to 1-inch. Place them with the parsnips in a small bowl. Set aside.

6. Heat a dutch oven or rondeau over medium heat and add the canola oil. Sear the chicken pieces two at a time, but don't crowd the pan. No need to cook them fully. Set aside on a clean plate when done with each piece.

🔔 If you are a good multi-tasker, you can sear the chicken and cut the vegetables at the same time. If not, don't stress, it's better to be focussed on one task at a time.

7. If the pan looks dry, add more oil. Add the onions and sauté for 3-5 minutes or until translucent. Add the garlic and ginger and sauté for an additional 1-2 minutes. Stir in 2 tablespoons of Ras el Hanout and cook for 1 minute.

8. Stir in the salt, tomato paste, chicken stock, and saffron.

9. Add the parsnips, potatoes, tomato quarters, and chicken. Ensure everything is below the liquid line, and nestle everything down if necessary. Bring to a simmer and cover. Set a timer for 30 minutes.

10. Mince the preserved lemon. Halve the olives and quarter the apricots. Add to the pot. If using lemon juice instead of preserved lemons, wait until the end to add it.

FINALE

1. Test the potatoes and parsnips for softness. Taste for salt and spice. If you did not use preserved lemon, add fresh lemon juice now. Tweak salt and lemon until it tastes balanced to you. You can add more Ras el Hanout, salt, olive juice, or a squeeze of fresh lemon. Remember to start small, taste, then increase.

2. Divide the couscous onto each plate and cover with Tagine, ensuring the chicken is evenly shared.

basic kids mac n cheese

BRUCE WALLIS 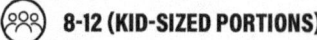 **30 MINUTES**   **8-12 (KID-SIZED PORTIONS)**   **VEGETARIAN**

Macaroni and cheese is a classic All-American dish that is loved by kids and grown-ups alike. Here we take the classic Kids Mac recipe served since "the beginning of time," as we say, and give it an adult spin. Make the Basic Kids Mac to please the young ones, but if you crave more excitement, the additional adult fixings include beer, cayenne pepper, and a crunchy topping. Consider leftovers a blessing. Portion, and then flatten extras in freezer bags (flat makes for faster defrosting). When reheating, add just a little milk, cream, or water to the pan. We all have nights when we want to pull a rabbit out of a hat!

gather

pasta pot, medium-sized sauce pot, liquid measuring cups, measuring spoons, whisk, box grater, silicon rubber spatula, pasta strainer

6 Tbsp organic butter

1 ½ cups organic heavy cream

1 ½ cups organic 2% milk

6 Tbsp all-purpose flour

1 tsp kosher salt

½ tsp onion powder

½ tsp garlic powder

⅛ tsp mustard powder

1 lb organic shredded cheese

1 lb cavatappi noodles or macaroni

1. Set 3-4 quarts of water on to boil.

2. Heat a saucepot over medium heat, add the butter and let it melt. Measure out the cream and milk. Set aside.

3. Whisk the flour into the butter until incorporated. Switch to a rubber spatula and continuously stir until the roux turns light brown.

4. Switch back to the whisk and slowly pour in the cream and milk. The roux will clump up, but continue whisking and pouring until smooth. Switch to the rubber spatula again and make sure there are no hidden spots of roux in the corners of the pot. If so, whisk them into the bechamel.

5. Whisk in the salt, onion powder, garlic powder, and mustard.

6. Bring to a gentle bubbling simmer. (The action of simmering the sauce triggers the thickening. Meaning the flour has begun to work its magic, transforming our milky potion into a thick bechamel base for our cheese sauce.)

7. Add about 1 tablespoon of salt to the boiling water. When it returns to a boil, add the pasta and stir. Have your strainer ready in the sink.

8. Lower the heat on the bechamel sauce to the lowest setting. Whisk in the cheese, one handful at a time. Wait until it is melted before adding more. If the cheese is slow to melt, turn up the heat a little. Continue until all the cheese is added to the sauce, then remove it from the heat.

9. When the pasta is al dente, strain it. Return the pasta to the cooking pot, but not on the hot burner. Pour the cheese sauce over the noodles. Use the rubber spatula to mix. Taste for salt, then dish it up to the kiddos! Or add the adult fixings...

recipe tip: Mix and match any variety of cheeses you like. I often take all my leftover bits of cheese and toss them in this recipe.

"adult" mac

BRUCE WALLIS **40 MINUTES (+30 MINUTES FOR BASIC KIDS MAC)**

The following bread crumb topping and beer slurry are just the beginning of what you can do with this dish! Start with the beer slurry, then add smoked salmon and pesto or crispy bacon and fresh tomatoes, carnitas meat & blanched broccoli, or black beans & salsa. You are only limited by your imagination.

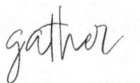 small saucepan, liquid measuring cup, measuring spoons, whisk, measuring cups and spoons, food processor or mixing bowl, chef knife and cutting board, sauté pan, spatula, glass baking pan or baking sheet, and oven-proof bowls

BEER STARTER

1- 12 oz can lager beer (PBR)

⅔ cup heavy cream

¼ tsp cayenne

½ tsp smoked paprika

1 tsp kosher salt

1 Tbsp + 1 ½ tsp dijon mustard

1 Tbsp honey

🔔 Start with your macaroni and cheese base. I recommend the Basic Kids Mac N Cheese which adds 30 minutes.

1. Combine everything in a saucepan over medium-high heat. Reduce to half volume.

BREAD CRUMB TOPPING

1 ½ cups Panko bread crumbs

¾ cup shredded Parmesan

5 Tbsp olive oil

1 tsp kosher salt

½ tsp smoked paprika

¼ tsp black pepper

¼ tsp ground bay leaves

¼ tsp granulated garlic

⅛ tsp cayenne pepper

⅛ tsp turmeric

1. Combine all the ingredients in a food processor. If you don't have one, chop the Parmesan to breadcrumb size, then combine everything in a mixing bowl. Note: if you don't have ground bay leaves, grind them in a clean coffee grinder. Also, if you like spicy foods, double the cayenne.

PUTTING IT TOGETHER

1. Turn the oven on to broil.

2. For each portion of mac and cheese, pour ¼ cup of the Beer Starter into a saucepan. Heat to a simmer, and add 2 cups of the Basic mac and cheese and any fillings. Be creative! Mix until combined and slightly bubbling around the edges.

3. You have two options. (1) For individual servings, put each portion into a bake-able bowl and top with the bread crumbs. This is best if each person wants different fillings. (2) For hot-dish family-style, place all the mixed mac into a baking pan and cover with the breadcrumbs. Either way, place the "Adult" Mac on the middle rack of the oven for 5-7 minutes or until golden brown.

original thai curry - chicken or tofu

CORY JOHNSON   🕐 **1 HOUR & 20 MINUTES**   👥 **SERVES 4**   ***VEGAN**   **DAIRY-FREE**

The Thai Curry is consistently among our highest sellers for a reason! Not only is this meal satisfying and nutritious, but it's also as versatile as your mood and the ingredients you have on hand. Make it with chicken, shrimp, tofu, or that bowl of steamed broccoli shunned by your kiddos. The recipe had not changed in twenty years, although recently it has been tweaked. Here it is in its original format for all the Curry lovers out there!

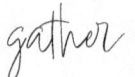 **large pot, 2 sauce pots, chef knife, cutting board, 1 large sauté pan or wok or 2 smaller sauté pans, measuring spoons and cups, mixing bowl, whisk, sauce pot, strainer**

RED CURRY SAUCE

1-13.5 oz cans coconut milk, full fat

1 Tbsp + 1 ½ tsp red curry paste

1 Tbsp g.f. tamari, or soy sauce

1 ½ tsp lemon juice

¼ tsp ground bay leaves or 2 whole leaves

1. Put all ingredients in a saucepot. Turn the heat to medium and whisk together. Simmer for approx. 10 minutes. The sauce will become darker, thicker, and reduced in volume. Taste for spiciness. Now is the time to add a bit more curry if you'd like. Turn off the heat and let it sit.

While filming an episode of 'Diners, Drive-In's, and Dives', at the Cafe, Guy Fieri leaned over and asked if we mixed the sesame seed oil with vegetable oil. "Of course!" was my reply.

There are two different types of sesame oil. One is toasted, darker, more pungent in taste, and often labeled as toasted sesame seed oil. The second is raw, lighter, mellower tasting and often labeled as sesame oil, omitting the word 'seed' or 'toasted'. However, these labeling rules are inconsistent. To distinguish the difference, look at the oil's color. In order to add the taste of sesame, choose the darker, toasted variety. Due to its strong taste, the general kitchen rule is to mix the dark/toasted style with vegetable oil. At the Cafe, we only purchased toasted sesame oil, which is why every recipe that lists sesame oil also has canola oil.

ENTRÉE

2 cups brown rice, medium or long grain

4 ½ cups water

2 cups broccoli florets (approx. 1 small head)

½ tray ice cubes

½ tsp fresh minced ginger

1 tsp fresh minced garlic

½ large zucchini, julienned

½ large red onion, julienned

1 large carrot, julienned

½ red pepper, julienned

1-2 Tbsp sesame seeds, toasted

12-16 oz chicken breast

1 pinch kosher salt

1 pinch granulated garlic

OR

1-14 oz pack extra firm tofu

1 tsp T&T Marinade 121 or g.f. tamari

2 Tbsp sesame and canola oil mixed

1-2 Tbsp mirin

1 bunch cilantro, de-stemmed

1 lime, wedged

1. Boil 4 ½ cups of water in a medium-sized pot. Add the rice, cover, and gently simmer until cooked, approx. 30 minutes.

2. Set 2 quarts of water on to boil.

3. Cut the broccoli into bite-sized florets. Half fill a deep bowl with ice cubes and cold water. Submerge the broccoli in the boiling water. When it turns bright green, in less than a minute, quickly strain the broccoli and plunge it into the ice water until cold. Strain and set aside. Note: You can skip this step if you want firm broccoli.

4. Peel and mince the garlic and ginger. Combine and set aside. Julienne the zucchini, red onion, carrot, and red pepper to about ¼-inch. Mix all the veggies together and set aside. See Julienne Tip 27 and 26 for tips about How much to Prep.

5. Dice the raw chicken or tofu into 1-inch cubes. Sprinkle the chicken with a pinch of salt and granulated garlic. Sprinkle the tofu with 1 teaspoon of T&T marinade or tamari. Wash your hands, cutting board, and knife.

6. Heat the sauté pan or wok over medium-high heat and add the sesame seeds. Stir and toast for 3-4 minutes. Remove them from the pan and set aside to cool.

7. Pour 1 tablespoon sesame/canola oil into the hot pan. When the oil is almost smoking hot, slide the chicken or tofu into the pan. Be careful of the splashing hot oil. Immediately jiggle the pan back and forth to prevent sticking. Sauté until the chicken is partially cooked or the tofu is crispy on each side. Note: If cooking chicken and tofu, use two pans here.

8. Add the vegetable mix and broccoli to the pan. Sauté for 5-7 minutes or until the pan shows caramelization, aka browning.

9. Add the ginger and garlic, and sauté for an additional 1-2 minutes.

10. Deglaze with mirin by pouring it along the outer rim of the pan.

11. Pour the Red Curry Sauce into the pan. Stir and let simmer until the sauce coats the vegetables and the chicken is fully cooked.

12. Divide the cooked rice onto four plates or bowls and pour a quarter of the curry onto each plate. Garnish with 1 teaspoon of sesame seeds on each plate, along with lime wedges and fresh cilantro.

recipe tips: You can prepare half tofu and half chicken easily as you will use two sauté pans.

If you don't have ground bay leaves, pulverize whole leaves in a clean coffee bean grinder. Alternatively, you can add 2-3 bay leaves while the sauce is simmering, then pull them out.

marathon meatballs

JILLIAN FORTE **1 HOUR & 30 MINUTES** **24 (2- 3 OZ MEATBALLS PER PERSON)** *GLUTEN-FREE *DAIRY-FREE

Every carnivore has to have a killer meatball recipe in their repertoire. These winning meatballs are a staple during our crazy-busy-carbo-loading Grandma's Marathon weekend. You can also find them served occasionally as a pasta special during the year. There are no strange or hard-to-find ingredients here. Mix up these tasty meatballs for some good old-fashioned comfort food and fuel to burn!

gather

small bowl, large mixing bowl, liquid measuring cup, measuring cups, measuring spoons, chef knife and cutting board, mesh strainer, baking sheets, mixing spoon, 2 or 3 oz scoop

1 small square ciabatta or 2 slices of sliced bread *sub g.f.

½ cup milk *sub water

½ lb bacon, diced

½ cup fresh minced parsley (approx. ½ bunch)

1 Tbsp fresh minced garlic

½ large yellow onion, minced

1 lb ground pork (Yker Acres)

1½ lbs ground chuck beef, any cut is suitable

1¾ tsp kosher salt

¾ tsp black pepper

¾ tsp red pepper flakes

¼ tsp + cayenne

1½ tsp dried basil

1½ tsp dried oregano

¾ tsp dried sage

½ cup shredded Parmesan

1 large egg

1. Heat the oven to 400°.

2. Crumble or tear the bread into a small bowl, cover with milk, and let soak.

3. Dice the bacon as small as possible. Note: Big chunks of bacon will stick out of the meatballs and cause them to crumble, cut them to less than ¼-inch. Cook over medium heat in a sauté pan until crunchy. Strain through a wire mesh strainer. Conversely, cook the strips, cool on a paper towel, then chop. Place the bacon bits into a large mixing bowl. Discard or reserve the fat. See Staff Tip 30.

4. De-stem and mince the parsley (discard, or save the stems for stock). Mince the garlic. Mince the onion to ¼-inch or smaller. Place in the mixing bowl.

5. Add all the remaining ingredients. Add more cayenne if you like spicy foods.

6. Strain the bread from the milk by pressing into a wire mesh strainer or squeezing by hand. Discard the milk and add the bread to the mix.

7. Line a baking sheet with either foil or parchment paper.

8. Mix the meatballs. This is best done with your hands to ensure every ingredient is fully incorporated. You will roll the meatballs with your hands later, so you may as well get dirty now.

9. Scoop the meat into approx. 20-24 3oz balls. If you want a precise size, you can use a meat/ice cream scoop.

10. Form the balls by rolling and compacting the meat between your palms. Ensure there are no clumps of onion, bacon, or bread that will cause the ball to split. Place them on the prepared baking sheet. Remember, the meatballs will shrink a little when cooked.

11. Bake for approximately 20-25 minutes. Cut one in half to make sure it is cooked all the way through. You may as well give it a little taste while you're at it! Any leftovers freeze wonderfully for a quick dinner later. See Freezing Tip 30.

🔔 This bake time is almost perfect for boiling pasta and warming up a simple sauce. Viola!

The legacy of Barb and Carla's Cafe comes from its longevity, and the love of them putting their own money, time, and effort into the place, and believing in it so much. They fostered a lot of people by giving them a livelihood that meant something. It enabled them to buy houses and do life. They made people happy, and that's just totally admirable. It was a precious place to work, play, and grow up. Carla's brother put it to her when she was opening the restaurant and she told him, "I can make a difference this way." - Sonja Helland (server)

I loved how loudly you could be yourself at the Cafe. There was a high level of peer respect, so people gave each other a lot of space to do their jobs in their own way. I always loved what a bunch of funny/struggling/thriving/silly/surprising/adventurous, and brave folks there were to talk to every day! And the food was good. It was the only restaurant job where I felt like the management and ownership had my back. I also had many wonderful regular customers that I miss seeing. Working at the Cafe rarely felt like work. - Sophie Gris (server)

rosemary cream
& butternut squash pasta

PETER RAVINSKI   **50 MINUTES**   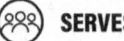 **SERVES 6**   ***GLUTEN-FREE**   **VEGETARIAN**

This late fall pasta bowl is one of my favorites. I love searching around my plate for the sweet yellow squash pieces or discovering a savory mushroom in the rosemary-infused cream sauce. A chunky sauce style like this invites stabbing with a fork and therefor works well with bite-sized noodle types. Try it over rotini, farfalle, or penne. Use twistable noodles like linguine and angel hair for sauces that are thin or slurp-able.

gather

chef knife, cutting board, mixing bowl, baking sheet, pasta pot, large sauté pan, liquid measuring cup, measuring spoons, measuring cups

4 cups diced butternut or buttercup squash, 1-inch

3 Tbsp olive oil

2 Tbsp kosher salt

½ + tsp black pepper

1 lb pasta, rigatoni, farfalle or penne *sub g.f. noodles

8 oz mushrooms, crimini, button or wild-harvested, ¼-inch sliced

2 Tbsp fresh minced shallot

1 ½ tsp fresh minced garlic

2 Tbsp white wine

1- 5.5 oz bag spinach, chopped

1 ½ cups heavy cream

1 ½ tsp fresh minced rosemary

1 cup shredded Parmesan

1. Heat the oven to 425°.

2. Peel, de-seed, and dice the squash into 1-inch cubes. See Recipe Tip 96.

3. Toss the squash cubes in 1 tablespoon olive oil. Sprinkle with ¼ teaspoon salt and a pinch of black pepper. Pour a little oil on the baking dish and rub it to coat before placing the squash. Bake for 15-20 minutes.

4. Set a pot of 4 quarts of water on to boil. Add 1+ tablespoon salt to the water. See Pro Tip on the following page.

5. Slice the mushrooms to ¼-inch and set aside. Mince the shallot and garlic, and set aside together. Rough chop the spinach and set aside. Mince the fresh rosemary. Mincing a little extra rosemary is OK. You can add it later if you'd like.

6. When the pasta water is boiling, pour the pasta in and give it an immediate stir. Set a timer according to the package.

7. Check the squash, pull the sheet pan out of the oven, and test one from the center of the pan to see if it is soft all the way through. Use a spatula to pry the pieces up and flip them over. If they need more time, give them a stir, pop them back in the oven and check at 5-minute intervals. Once fully cooked, set aside.

8. Heat the sauté pan over medium and add 2 tablespoons of olive oil. Once the pan is hot, sauté the mushrooms for 4-5 minutes, stirring occasionally, until just brown. Add the shallot and garlic and cook for 1-2 minutes.

9. Deglaze the pan with the white wine by pouring it around the rim. Cook for 1 minute. Add the heavy cream, rosemary and 1 teaspoon salt, ½ teaspoon black pepper and give it a good stir. Let the cream come up to a simmer and reduce by a quarter. Taste the sauce, you can easily add more salt or rosemary now.

10. Scrape the baked squash pieces into the sauté pan and stir.

11. Strain the pasta, letting it sit in the strainer over the pot, which is removed from the heat source. Note: Do not run water over the pasta or coat it with oil. We want the sauce to grab onto the noodles.

12. Once the sauce has reduced, add the spinach. As soon as the leaves wilt, turn off the heat.

13. Put the pasta noodles back into the cooking pot. Pour in the sauce. Stir to combine. Taste one last time. Note: When pasta is cooked in salty water, it absorbs some salt, thus you will need less in the sauce. However, if none or not enough was added to the water, you may need to add more at this step. Keep in mind that the Parmesan is also salty.

14. Divide the pasta into 4 wide bowls and top with Parmesan cheese.

recipe tip: Trim both ends of the squash. Halve the squash, cutting the rounded bottom from the thinner top. Stand the narrow half of the squash upright and slice its skin off with a knife, or use a sharp vegetable peeler. Slice the top half lengthwise, creating 4-5 paddle-shaped pieces. Lay them flat, cut into 1-inch thick strips, then dice. For the rounded bottom, cut it in half. Use a sharp-edged spoon to scoop out the seeds. Peel with a vegetable peeler, then cut the flesh into strips and dice.

pro tip

"Proper pasta water is important. You want a lot of it and it should be saltier than you'd think. If you've ever gone swimming in the ocean and gotten a mouthful, that's the taste to aim for. Use less salt when boiling potatoes. They will absorb a lot more of the salt than pasta will."
- Ben Butter (line cook)

shrimp, scallop & chorizo paella

JILLIAN FORTE **1 HOUR & 45 MINUTES** **SERVES 4-5**   **GLUTEN-FREE**   **DAIRY-FREE**

Anyone who has eaten traditional Paella knows the multi-layered joys of this Spanish dish, the comradery of people sharing a piping-hot paella pan, the myriad of regional seafood and meats, and the crunchy rice on the bottom that seems to have absorbed and crystallized the flavors. I will be the first to admit that the genuine experience of Spanish paella is difficult to replicate, but it is worth the effort! In Spain, they commonly use bomba rice. I've found a suitable substitute in short-grain, white basmati. Though most of us don't have a classic paella pan, a large cast iron pan works well. Note that in this recipe, the rice is cooked separately, a restaurant step that makes for speedier ticket times. Cooking the shrimp, scallops, and chorizo in the pan and then adding the rice and sofrito mimics the traditional layered flavor. Oh, and remember to let the rice get a little crunchy on the bottom. It's called socarrat, most Spaniards consider that the best part!

gather   **heavy-bottomed pot, measuring spoons and cups, rubber spatula, chef knife and cutting board, food processor, mesh strainer, 2 sauce pots, large & deep cast iron pan or rondeau**

recipe tip: I have experimented with this dish, using regular roasted red peppers instead of Piquillo peppers, and wow! Make the effort to find the Piquillo.

GOLDEN RICE

2 Tbsp canola oil

2 tsp turmeric

1 tsp ground cumin

3 cups white rice, short-grained basmati, or Bomba

6 cups water

1 Tbsp kosher salt

10+ strands saffron

1 Tbsp lemon juice

1. Heat a heavy-bottomed pot over medium heat and add 2 tablespoons of olive oil. Stir in the turmeric and cumin, and bloom for 1-2 minutes.

2. Add the rice. Stir and fry for 4-5 minutes, or until it turns slightly opaque. Some browning of the rice will occur.

3. Add the water, salt, and saffron. Stir only once to even out the rice. Bring to a boil, then lower the heat. Simmer most of the water off, approx. 10 minutes.

   🔔 Start the Saffron Sofrito.

4. Cover, turn off the heat, and let the steam and residual heat continue to cook the rice, approx. 20 minutes.

5. Squeeze the lemon juice over the rice. Fluff the rice with a fork while checking it to ensure it is done. If not, re-cover and let sit until cooked.

pro tip

Heat a cast iron pan on the stove over medium-high heat. Add 1-2 tablespoons oil or clarified butter. Swirl the oil around in the pan until you see the first indication of smoke. Wipe the interior of the pan with a paper towel to coat the entire surface with a thin layer of oil. Reduce heat to keep just below the smoke point. Add more oil and repeat the process 1-2 more times. This temporarily seasons the pan. The oil becomes baked onto the metal, smoothing the surface, and keeping food from sticking to the pan. Great for omelets! - Benjamin Zaban-Boylan (line cook)

SAFFRON SOFRITO

¼ medium yellow onion, chopped

¼ cup piquillo peppers, chopped

1 small tomato, diced

1 large clove garlic, chopped

1 Tbsp olive oil

⅛ tsp smoked paprika

1 pinch ground fennel seed

1 pinch ground rosemary

½ tsp sea salt or kosher

2 Tbsp white wine

2 cups chicken stock 145

6 shrimp shells
(from peeling the shrimp)

5-10 strands saffron

1. Rough chop the onion, ¼ cup piquillo peppers, tomato, and 1 large garlic clove. Blend in a food processor or blender until smooth. If you don't have a food processor, mince the onion, pepper, and garlic, and dice the tomato.

2. Heat a small pot over medium-high heat, and add the olive oil. Add the vegetables and sauté for 5-8 minutes. You want it fully cooked, however, it's difficult to discern once the vegetables are pureed. Notice the sharp scent of raw onions when you start. Cook until the smell has mellowed to almost sweet.

3. Stir in the dry spices and cook for 1 minute.

4. Pour in the wine and cook for 1 minute. Add the chicken stock and saffron.

5. Peel the shrimp from the shells. See Peeling Shrimp Tip 29. Place half of the shells into the pot (discard or freeze the remaining shells for stock). Put the shrimp into a small bowl and sprinkle with a pinch of salt and a pinch of smoked paprika.

6. Simmer the sofrito until reduced by less than half, approx. 30 minutes.

🔔 Start preparing the finale.

7. Pour the sofrito through a fine wire strainer. Discard the pulp and reserve the stock.

FINALE

12 oz jar Piquillo peppers, minus previously used

2 links chorizo
(Yker Acres)

8-12 scallops

12-16 shell-on shrimp, peeled

1-2 Tbsp olive oil

1 pinch kosher salt

1 pinch smoked paprika

1 cup peas, fresh or frozen

1 lemon

1. Slice the remaining Piquillo peppers into long strips and set aside. Slice the chorizo sausage into ¼-inch circles, and set aside. De-foot each scallop by pulling off the little attached lump. Discard the foot. Set the scallops aside.

2. Heat the cast iron pan over medium heat and add cooking olive oil. Cook the chorizo until almost crunchy. Remove and set aside. Reuse the oily pan for the next step.

3. Cook the scallops and shrimp for approx. 2 minutes per side. Do not overcook. Remove and set aside.

4. Fill the pan with the cooked rice and pat it flat. Place the pepper slices on top like the spokes of a wheel. Scatter the chorizo, shrimp, scallops, and peas on top.

5. Pour half the saffron sofrito around the edges of the pan. Drizzle the other half over the rice and meats and let simmer. If the rice was cold, cover the pan for 5 minutes. Cook until the bottom of the rice is getting crunchy. You may need to spin the pan to cook evenly, depending on the vagaries of your stovetop.

6. Halve the lemon and use a fork to remove any visible seeds.

7. Set the cast iron pan on a coaster at the dinner table. Squeeze the fresh lemon over the dish for a dramatic table-side presentation.

minnesota wild rice, white fish & roasted root vegetables

MICAH NEWMAN **1 HOUR & 40 MINUTES** **SERVES 4** ***GLUTEN-FREE**

Nothing says Minnesota more than manoomin and fresh-caught fish! We like to source Lake Superior Whitefish for the restaurant, but the recipe works well with many types of fish. These pairings are my autumn favorite. The creamy wild rice, sautéed fish, and roasted root vegetables, are grounding and comforting. In spring, substitute grilled asparagus, or sautéed ramps, with a splash of white wine.

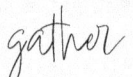 two mixing bowls, chef knife & cutting board, liquid measuring cup, measuring cups, measuring spoons, zester, rubber spatula, wax or parchment paper, aluminum foil, baking sheet, saucepan, heavy-bottomed pot, wide plate, sauté pan, fish spatula

ROASTED ROOT VEGETABLES

1 medium beet or 2 small

¼ rutabaga, 1-inch dice

1 medium carrot, 1-inch dice

1 medium parsnip, 1-inch dice

1 small turnip, 1-inch dice

5 tsp canola oils

salt & pepper, to taste

1-2 Tbsp fresh minced herbs (use 2 or more of any type)

1 Tbsp salted butter

1. Lightly grease a baking sheet. Heat the oven to 425°.

   🔔 If you are preparing the entire dish, and haven't softened the butter, do so now. Place the butter in a bowl near the warming stove.

2. Cut the tops and tails off the beets. Place them in the middle of a piece of aluminum foil. Cover with 1 teaspoon canola oil, wrap and place in the oven. These will take the longest, so it's best to start with them. Set a timer for 1 hour. They may take an additional 30 minutes, depending on their size.

3. Peel then cut the rutabaga into approx. 1-inch cubes. Place into a mixing bowl and add 1 teaspoon of cooking oil and a pinch of salt and pepper. Toss and mix. Lay this on the lightly greased baking sheet, off to one side. Repeat with the parsnips, carrots, and turnips. Keep each vegetable separate. Note: Each root vegetable has a slightly different baking time. Keeping them apart allows you to remove a fully cooked vegetable from the baking sheet while leaving the rest to continue cooking.

4. Place the root vegetables in the oven and set a timer for 30 minutes.

   🔔 Move on to the compound butter and wild rice.

5. When all the vegetables are fork-able soft, put them in a mixing bowl.

6. Place 1 tablespoon of butter in the bowl to melt. Mince 2 tablespoons of herbs. (If you are preparing the compound butter, mince 3+ tablespoons and set aside the extra.) Toss together and set on the stovetop to keep warm while the beets finish.

7. Test the beets when the 1-hour timer goes off. They are done when a paring knife slides in easily. If not done, add another 10-15 minutes. Cool beets just enough to handle by placing them in the fridge for 15 minutes. Peel and hopefully the skins will slide off. Then dice into 1-inch cubes and add to the other root vegetables, toss to combine. Taste for salt.

COMPOUND BUTTER

1+ Tbsp fresh minced herbs (use 2 or more of any type)

½ lemon

6 Tbsp salted butter, softened (⅔ stick)

1. Mince the herbs (if you haven't already) and place 1+ tablespoons into the softened butter in the bowl. Zest the lemon and add half the zest to the butter. Cut the lemon into quarters and juice one wedge of the lemon into the bowl (reserve half of the zest and the remaining quarters for the wild rice). Mix with a rubber spatula.

2. Place a large piece of wax paper, parchment paper, or plastic wrap on the table. Spoon the prepared butter onto the sheet. Use the spatula to form the butter into a 1-inch thick log. Take the long side of the sheet and fold it over the butter log. Gently roll the butter to even its shape using your fingers as needed. Tightly twist the ends of the sheet to seal in the butter. Refrigerate until firm.

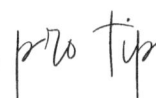
pro tip

Compound butter is one of those chefs' secrets that both wastes not and enhances. It's a great way to preserve surplus herbs, and having it on hand, fresh or frozen, can make an "I don't want to cook" meal into something special. Just melt a slice over steamed veggies, rice, or noodles!

WILD RICE RISOTTO

1 cup water

2 cups chicken stock

2 tsp canola oil

¾ cup finely diced yellow onion (approx. ½)

1 ½ tsp fresh minced garlic

1 cup wild rice, MN or WI grown

6 Tbsp white wine

1 ½ tsp kosher salt

3 Tbsp fresh minced parsley

¼ cup heavy cream

3 Tbsp grated Parmesan

¼ lemon

1. Add the water and stock to a saucepan and bring to a gentle simmer.

2. Peel and finely dice the onion, measure, then set aside. Mince the garlic and set aside.

3. Heat a heavy-bottomed pot over medium heat, and add the oil. Sauté the onion until soft, approx. 4 minutes. Add the garlic and cook for one minute. Add the wild rice and cook for 2-3 minutes.

4. Deglaze the pot with the white wine. Add the salt.

5. Add 1-2 ladles of the hot stock-water mix to the rice and constantly stir. Once the liquid is absorbed, add another 1-2 ladles. Repeat until all the liquid is absorbed into the rice. The rice should be soft and split open. If not, add more stock or water and continue cooking.

6. Add the heavy cream and Parmesan. Lower the heat and stir until the Parmesan has melted.

7. Turn off the heat. Add the reserved lemon zest. Juice one reserved lemon wedge into the rice. Stir, taste, and add more salt or lemon juice if needed.

8. Mince and stir in the fresh parsley.

SEASONED FLOUR

¾ cup all-purpose flour
*sub rice flour

1 Tbsp Old Bay seasoning

1 ½ tsp kosher salt

1 ¼ tsp ground coriander

1 ¼ tsp black pepper

1 tsp smoked paprika

1. Mix all spices with the flour, and stir well to combine.

2. Lay out about 1 cup of Seasoned Flour onto a plate, and set aside. Cut one ¼-inch thick disk of compound butter for each filet and set aside.

FINALE

4 Whitefish filets (8-9 oz) skinned and de-boned

1 Tbsp salted butter

1 lemon, wedged

1. Ensure that your fish filets are free from bones by laying them on your cutting board and running your fingers over the flesh. If you feel something poking you, slice the bones out. See Channel Method Pro Tip 68.

2. Melt the plain butter in a sauté pan over medium heat. Dredge 2 pieces of fish in the seasoned flour. When the butter is bubbling, place the floured fish in the pan. Immediately jiggle the pan so the fish doesn't stick. Cook the filets until golden brown, flip and repeat. Lay the fish filets on a plate. Place a disk of compound butter on top of each. Repeat this step with the remaining filets.

3. Place the Wild Rice Risotto on the corner of each plate. Next, add the Roasted Root Vegetables near the rice, and place one golden buttered fish filet slightly on top of the rice. Serve with lemon wedges.

I know that Barb and Carla are trying to do good things for all of us here. I feel like I've got a support system here if I really need it. - Shelly Berry (server)

I recall all the years I was working so tirelessly to feed people, longing for validation that I was creating things that people would love. I learned over time that not only was I able to create many amazing dishes; I could do it in a way that was nourishing, comforting, and special in every way. I truly found myself during my time At Sara's Table. I became a much more well-rounded chef; I learned the importance of family, how to care for the people I love through food, and to respect our earth and all it provides. Sara's Table was a huge part of my growth, both in my career and my personal life. I wouldn't be as successful as I am today without the experience I had in that kitchen. - Channie McCall (line cook)

I worked with a ragtag band of misfits whose passion for the culinary arts to this day remains unsurpassed by any others I have witnessed. The fires burn, the scars remain, and the offerings were pure. We sweat. We laughed. We loved. Oh.. and XXX... thank you, Heather ;) - Jackie Fontaine (prep cook)

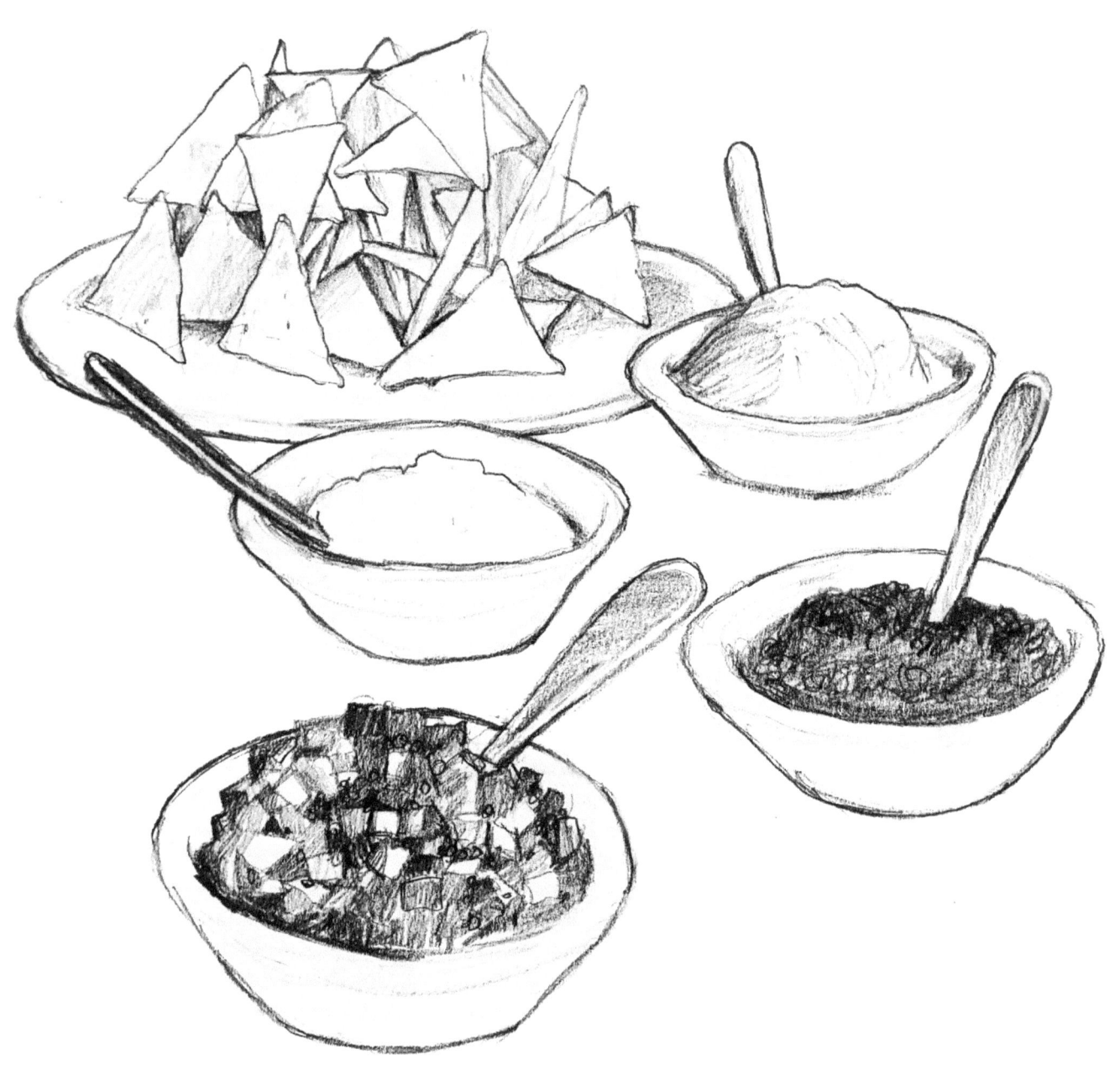

ILLUSTRATED BY: BENJAMIN ZABAN-BOYLAN *(LINE COOK)*

small plates, sauces, & sides

Classically, chefs compose complete meals with a protein, a starch, and a vegetable, while relishing the infinite combinations! As a former vegetarian who spent years eating sides at family feasts, I learned that a great side dish often steals the meal. These recipes are some of my absolute favorites from the Cafe.

This section's recipes will inspire your meal planning and add zing to your table. Jeremy's Pico de Gallo blows other salsas out of the water. My mouth waters just thinking about Matt's Kimchi. I never knew Brussels sprouts were snack-able until Natalie introduced me to this recipe's method. Included here are comforting potatoes, lively rice, and more than one potluck party winner. I've also added an introduction to smoking salmon, a savory marinade for tofu and tempeh, and a foolproof method for hard-boiled eggs. This section is full of hidden gems!

additional sides in other chapters:

bright green basil pesto

HEATHER ERICKSON 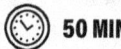 50 MINUTES 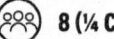 8 (¼ CUP PORTIONS)   **GLUTEN-FREE**   **VEGETARIAN**   **KETO**

If you love the smoked salmon omelet at the Cafe, here's how to make its delicious accompanying pesto. The color, freshness, and multidimensional flavors of this sauce are nothing short of inspirational. Even in winter, the smell of this pesto will elicit thoughts of a garden bursting with potential, evoke warm nights on the patio with a sweating glass of chardonnay, and a cool breeze off the lake. Huzzah Heather!

gather

4 mixing bowls, small strainer, chef knife, cutting board, liquid measuring cup, measuring cups, measuring spoons, scale, food processor

1 oz fresh basil leaves (2- 1 oz small clam shells packs)

2 cups parsley, de-stemmed (approx. 1 bunch curly leaf)

10 oz spinach (1¼- 8oz bags)

¾ tsp kosher salt

1 tsp fresh minced garlic

¼ cup slivered almonds

1 Tbsp pine nuts

¾ cup shredded Parmesan

¾ cup + 2 Tbsp extra virgin olive oil

½ lemon

1. De-stem the basil and place it in a bowl. De-stem and measure the parsley. Add to the bowl. Set spinach in a second bowl.

2. Put the salt, minced garlic, almonds, pine nuts, and Parmesan in a 3rd bowl. You can lightly toast the almonds and pine nuts, but it is unnecessary.

3. Measure the oil. Juice half a lemon into the oil. See Lemon Juicing Tip 27. Note: You will have 3 bowls and spinach ready to go.

4. Put about ¼ - ½ cup of the nut mix into the food processor or blender. Process until the nuts are chopped, less than 30 seconds. Add a small handful of herbs, 2 handfuls of spinach, and some of the oil/juice mixture. Puree until smooth. If the blades won't pull in the leaves, stop the machine, scrape down the sides and add 1-2 tablespoons of oil/juice. Once smooth, pour into a 4th bowl.

5. Repeat the previous step until all your ingredients are blended and poured into the 4th bowl. It doesn't matter if you end up with a lot of spinach in the last batch or if you run out of the nut mix by the second round. It's all going to be blended in the bowl. So blend, pour and, at the end, mix it up!

6. Taste the pesto. Warning, it is so yummy you risk green teeth all day! Add salt, oil, or lemon juice if needed.

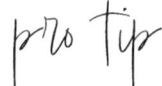

pro tip

This recipe makes a lot of pesto, so freeze any leftovers. Label 3-4 small zip-top bags with the date and contents, using a sharpie. Roll the zipper of the bag down once or twice (this prevents pesto from gumming up the zip). Use a ½ or ¼ cup measuring cup to scoop and portion the pesto into the bags. Seal and freeze.

pico de gallo

JEREMY BARANY **20 MINUTES**   **6 (½ CUP PORTIONS)**   **GLUTEN-FREE**   **VEGAN**   **DAIRY-FREE**

This Pico de Gallo is well worth the prep time and will outshine any store-bought salsa! Fresh, tangy, and healthy, it is the defining ingredient of our amazing breakfast tacos. There is a lot of knife work involved, and the smaller the dice, the better. So sharpen your blade, watch your fingertips, and enjoy the process. Try this wonderful Pico on scrambled eggs, nachos, or straight-up with corn chips.

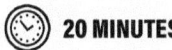

chef knife, cutting board, mixing bowl, zester, measuring spoons

3 large Beefsteak tomatoes, de-seeded, ¼-inch dice

1 cup red onion, finely diced (approx. 1 small)

½ cup minced cilantro (approx. ½ bunch)

1 jalapeño, minced

1 large lime

¾ tsp kosher salt

1. De-seed and dice the tomato to ¼-inch. Place in a mixing bowl. Knife not cutting the tomato? See the two Tomato Tips 29.

2. Finely dice the onions, the smaller the better. See Onions, finely diced 27 for Jillian's method. Add to the bowl.

3. De-stem the cilantro, then chiffonade or mince. Add to the bowl. See Chiffonade Tip 25.

4. De-seed and mince the jalapeño, use a disposable glove if possible. Add to the bowl.

5. Zest the lime into the bowl. Roll the lime on the counter while pressing firmly. Cut the lime in half and juice it into the bowl.

6. Add the salt and mix everything. Adjust to your preference.

I love it here. Carla's great. They treat me well. As a cook, I have freedom, and I get to experiment. Everyone's chill, and in a good mood all the time - Jeremy Barany (line cook)

harissa aioli

BRUCE WALLIS **1 HOUR & 15 MINUTES** **SERVES 10 (¼ CUP PORTIONS)** **GLUTEN-FREE** ***VEGAN**

Harissa aioli has made frequent appearances at the Cafe since Bruce first put it on the menu to accompany the Chester Wedges, our sliced and fried baked potatoes. It started as Harissa sauce, a Tunisian hot pepper paste full of aromatics (garlic, caraway, and coriander) before morphing into a mayonnaise. The restaurant goes through it with ferocity, featuring it on burgers, as a side, or as a smear. This recipe makes a fair amount, but it will refrigerate for 2-3 weeks. And don't worry, you'll probably eat it long before that!

gather

pot, Vitamix or blender, measuring spoons, measuring cups, spatula, squeeze bottle or jar

3-4 dried New Mexico peppers

3-4 dried Guajillo peppers

2+ Tbsp soaking water

2 cloves garlic, peeled

2 tsp extra virgin olive oil

½ tsp kosher salt

½ tsp ground caraway

½ tsp ground cumin

½ tsp ground coriander

2 cups mayonnaise (Hellmans)
*sub Vegan Aioli 55

1. Crack open each pepper and place them together in a small pot. Cover with water and bring to a boil. Turn off the heat and let the water cool down for about 30 minutes. Save the soaking water for steps 2 and 3.

2. De-stem and de-seed the peppers. Discard the stem and seeds. Note: Dunk the peppers in the soaking water to remove loosened seeds.

3. Blend the peppers, garlic cloves, olive oil, and 2+ tablespoons of the soaking water in a kitchen blender or Vitamix. Process until the pepper pieces are less than ⅛-inch.

4. Add the salt, dried spices, and mayonnaise. Blend until the pepper pieces are indiscernible and the aioli is a uniform color. Pour into a squeeze bottle or place in a labeled jar.

Carla is the most caring person you will ever meet. She is so welcoming and whole-hearted about everything. Working at the Cafe was probably one of the greatest times of my life. It was a lot of fun. I met a lot of people who have stuck around in my life. A lot of impactful people.
— Jenny (Pilcher) Quinn (barista)

I loved Barb and Carla, their mission, and the clientele. I liked being a part of the neighborhood community aspect. I worked there for almost 14 years. It's a long time and has been my longest-held job to date. I took pride in the Cafe. I was able to buy my first house and build a little equity, which allowed me to do the things I am working on now, which is Lake Superior Brewing Company. I always felt like Barb and Carla genuinely saw me and cared about my well-being. They supported me through a time when, as women, we shouldn't have to worry about taking off 6 weeks of unpaid leave. - Sarah Maxim (server)

Fans of the bar may remember the drinks named after popular servers. There was the "Sonja Smash" (Sonja Helland), the "Sassy Ellen" (Ellen Vaagen), "Red's Baby" (Sarah Runholt-Farrell), and "Melissa's Manhattan" (Melissa Weisser)

matt's kimchi

MATT LINDBERG 1 HOUR + 3-9 DAYS 1-GALLON JAR **GLUTEN-FREE** **VEGAN** **DAIRY-FREE**

I have tried numerous Kimchi recipes over the years, in search of a flavor that resonated with me. I even tried one written in Korean with the help of Google translate. All of my attempts ended with so-so results. One day my friend Matt Lindberg, who had spent a year in Korea, let me try his version. It was mouth-wateringly fantastic! He agreed to let me use his recipe at the Cafe, as long as I gave him credit. I never got his name on the menu. Here's to you Matt, many thanks!

Since kimchi is fermented, you need to take some precautions. Use a sanitized jar and disposable rubber gloves so you don't inadvertently add bacteria to your batch. Ferment the kimchi away from fresh fruits and vegetables, as they can be a source of airborne contamination. Lastly, Kimchi needs to ferment until it reaches a pH of 4.2 or lower. At the Cafe, we use a pH tester (pH papers won't work). If you don't have one, your taste buds will suffice. Begin tasting your kimchi on day 3 or 4. If it tastes like salty vegetables, it is not yet ready. The flavor should be a sour that makes your mouth water, but not pucker. There should never be white or black mold growing on it. If by days 7 to 9, your kimchi doesn't seem right, start over. As kitchen folx say "When in doubt, throw it out!"

gather

scale, disposable gloves (optional), chef knife, cutting board, box grater, large bowl or pot, small mixing bowl, long-handled spoon, 1-gallon glass jar, pint glass, cheesecloth, rubber band

4.5 lbs napa cabbage (approx. 3-4 heads)

3 Tbsp kosher salt

2.5 oz carrot, shredded (approx. 2 medium)

1.5 oz fresh minced ginger (approx. 2-3-inch piece)

2 oz fresh minced garlic (approx. 3 large cloves)

2 oz green onion, ⅛-inch discs (approx. 1 bunch)

2 oz red onion (approx. ½ onion)

2 tsp cayenne

2 tsp gochugaru or an additional 1 tsp cayenne

1. Remove any brown leaves from the napa. Cut in half lengthwise. Rinse the inside to remove any dirt or sand. See FYI below. Let drip dry while you peel, then weigh out the other vegetables.

2. Shred the carrot on a box grater, then set it in a small bowl. Mince the garlic and ginger. Add to the bowl. See Ginger Tip 54.

3. Slice the green onion into ⅛-inch or thinner circles. Add to the bowl. Finely dice the red onion and add to the bowl. See Onions, finely minced 27 for Jillian's method.

4. Cut the root out of the cabbage with a V-shaped cut. Turn the cabbage so the cut side is on the board, then slice the cabbage ¼ - ½-inch thick starting on the leafy side. When you get to the last 2 inches, flip it wide side down and continue slicing. Put the cabbage into a large bowl or stock pot.

5. Sprinkle the salt onto the cabbage and massage it by squeezing and mixing the cabbage with your hands (I have even given it little punches when my fingers get tired). You are breaking down the cell walls of the cabbage, allowing the salt to penetrate. The volume will shrink as water is released. Keep massaging until the cabbage is submerged. Do not add water. If it doesn't seem wet enough at the end of about 5 minutes, don't worry. It will release more liquid as it ferments.

6. Pour the bowl of diced vegetables into the cabbage.

7. Add the spices. Note: this heat is a little above "Minnesota Nice". If you are spice weary, subtract some cayenne. Wait and see how the finished product comes out. Add more cayenne at that point.

8. Mix with a long-handled spoon or your hands.

9. Pack the vegetables and the liquid into your fermentation jar. Take a pint glass and fill it ¾ with water. Place inside the jar as a weight to keep the vegetables below the liquid line. The glass will protrude from the jar. If the liquid in the fermentation jar is near the top, put a plate beneath it to catch any spillover. Cover the glass jar and pint glass with a double-layered cheesecloth. Secure with a rubber band. Place in a location away from fresh fruits and veggies. The top of the fridge is a warm place that will speed the process along.

10. Taste test the kimchi on day three (the kimchi is usually finished on that day). However, it can take up to seven days to finish fermenting. Start tasting it on day three, then every day to follow its progress. When it has reached your preferred level of sourness, remove the pint glass and cover the jar with a lid and refrigerate. As long as the liquid covers the kimchi, it can last up to 3 months.

recipe tip: Some people prefer spring water for rinsing vegetables they will ferment, citing chlorinated water as a deterrent to the growth of good bacteria. Use purified water if so inclined. At the restaurant, we used tap water and had no problems.

pro tip

If you don't have a scale at home, use the one at the grocery store! Remember to round up though, particularly with the cabbage as the outside layers and root will be composted.

Carla and Barb are lovely people. They were always giving homeless employees free housing. We had an abusive boyfriend situation, and they said "you have that house right there next to the Cafe as long as you need." They were always like that. - Colleen Betts (head chef)

potato parsnip puree

NATALIE ALLESEE **55 MINUTES** **5 (1-2 CUP POTIONS)** **GLUTEN-FREE** **VEGETARIAN**

This puree is perfect for Thanksgiving dinner, or anytime you're craving comfort food. It's simple, but the method matters. Over-whipping potatoes give them a "gluey" texture, as Natalie would say. Gently mash and mix, then push through a strainer, or spin briefly in a food mill. Light and fluffy potatoes are the goal.

large pot, sauce pot, vegetable peeler, cheesecloth, food mill or firm cone strainer, spatula

1 gallon water

3 Tbsp +1 ¼ tsp kosher salt, divided

2 lbs russet potatoes, peeled and chopped

½ lb parsnips, peeled, 1-inch chop (approx. 1-2)

2 cups heavy cream

2 ½ tsp lemon juice

1 sprig fresh rosemary or 2 Tbsp dried whole

1 Tbsp black peppercorns

1. Boil the water, add 3 tablespoons of the salt, and return to a rolling boil.

2. Peel and rough chop the potatoes. Carefully place in the boiling water. Simmer until the potatoes are soft to the center.

3. Peel and chop the parsnips into approximately 1-inch chunks. Put in the sauce pot. Add the cream, lemon juice, and 1 ¼ teaspoon salt. Turn the heat to medium-high, bring to a low boil, then reduce the heat to medium.

4. Place the rosemary and peppercorns in the middle of the cheesecloth. Roll, and tie the ends together. Nestle the sachet into the parsnip pot. Cover and simmer until the parsnips are soft, about 20 minutes.

5. Strain the softened potatoesand set aside. If you are going to reheat the puree at a later time, then cooling them completely will help the final steps. Spread the potatoes on a baking pan and refrigerate. If serving immediately, cool at room temp until touchable.

6. Test the parsnips. They are done when easily pierced with a fork. Press the sachet against the side of the pot with the fork to get all the flavor and cream out. Discard.

7. Using a potato masher, mash the parsnips in the pot until pulpy.

8. If the potatoes are completely cooled, run them through a ricer. If they are warm, use the potato masher to get them as smooth as possible.

9. Combine the parsnips and potatoes and mix well with the potato masher or wooden spoon. You can serve the dish now or try the next step for a creamier texture.

10. Set a firm cone strainer over a clean pot or bowl. Push 1-2 cups of the potato-parsnip mixture through the strainer using a rubber spatula. Repeat with all the puree. Note: This method, though slightly tedious, removes lumps and yields a creamier puree. Do not use an immersion blender, food processor, or stand mixer. Each results in a gooey glop of potatoes, especially if the potatoes are hot.

seared brussels sprouts

NATALIE ALLESEE  **15 MINUTES** **SERVES 4 (1 CUP PORTIONS)**   **GLUTEN-FREE**   **VEGAN**   **DAIRY-FREE**

If you disavow Brussels sprouts, you've not tasted this preparation. The sear, bordering on burnt, creates the magic of this dish. This rough treatment transforms the bitter edge often associated with brassicas into a snack-worthy treat.

gather

heavy-bottomed pot or rondeau, chef's knife, cutting board, measuring cups, measuring spoons

4 cups Brussels sprouts, trimmed and halved

1 Tbsp canola oil

1 tsp kosher salt

½ tsp black pepper

2 Tbsp cider vinegar

1. Remove any blemished outer leaves on the Brussels sprouts and trim off the brown stem. Slice in half, through the root, so they stay intact.

2. Heat a heavy-bottomed pot, or rondeau on medium-high and add the cooking oil. Lay the Brussels sprouts in the pan cut side down. If they don't all fit, cook the sprouts in two batches, and divide the salt, pepper, and vinegar.

3. Sear the Brussels sprouts until they are dark brown on the bottom. You may need to move the pan around on the stovetop so each piece gets dark. They taste best, almost burnt!

4. Sprinkle them with salt and pepper.

5. Pour in the vinegar and quickly cover to steam the sprouts. Turn off the heat and wait 4-5 minutes.

6. Remove the lid and stir, dispersing the salt and pepper.

7. Pop one in your mouth to taste and serve the rest or repeat starting with step 3 with any remaining sprouts.

For years Sarah the Red (Runholt-Farrell) worked at the Cafe as either a server or the Front of House manager. Sometimes she would wait on guests that would lean in conspiratorially and ask if she was 'The Sara' of At Sara's Table? She laughed at first, but as the years went by, she would simply point to her name tag and the obvious H at the end of her name.

chevre potato tarts

ROLF HOLVIK 50 MINUTES (+ OPTIONAL 30 MINUTES) SERVES 4 (2 TARTS EACH)   GLUTEN-FREE   VEGETARIAN

Though not exactly heart-healthy, this side dish is divine! Use chevre, or substitute with a cheese of your choice. At the Cafe, we made impressive star-shaped tarts by overlapping thin layers of potato. For those who want this lovely presentation, I have included the star process at the end of the recipe. Be forewarned, they take time to learn. You might waste some potatoes, but the result will be dazzling.

2-24 hours ahead: Heat the oven to 450°. Bake 3 russet potatoes for approximately 40 minutes or until a knife slides through the center easily. Cool completely.

gather **baking sheet pan, paring knife, grater, mixing bowl, mixing spoon, chef's knife, cutting board, sauté pan, scale, measuring spoons, mandolin (optional)**

CHEVRE POTATOES

4 ½ cups shredded cooked russet potatoes (approx. 3-4)

½ cup yellow onion, minced

1 tsp fresh minced garlic

½ cup salted butter (1 stick)

8 oz chevre (2 small logs) **or cheese of choice**

2 Tbsp fresh sliced chives or 2 tsp fresh minced rosemary or sage

1 tsp kosher salt

¼ tsp white pepper

1. Peel the cooked potatoes with a paring knife. Shred on a box grater. Measure then set in a mixing bowl.

2. Mince the onions and garlic. Set aside separately. Slice the chives.

3. Melt the butter in a sauté pan over medium-low heat. Add the onions and sweat until translucent. Add the garlic and cook for an additional minute.

4. Crumble the chevre over the potatoes. Pour the hot onions and butter over the potatoes.

5. Add the chives, salt, and pepper and mix completely.

6. Form the potato mixture into 8 patties. Flatten each to approx. ¾ - 1-inch thickness. You can make the mix and patties 1 to 3 days in advance and hold them in the fridge. However, you need to form the patties while the cheese is warm and soft. Note: If you're making the Potato Skin Stars skip the next two steps for now.

COOK THE TARTS

1. Reheat the onion pan. There should be some residual butter. If not, add 2 teaspoons and let it melt. The pan needs to be hot to prevent sticking. Place the potato patties (or stars) in the pan, not touching. Cook until golden.

2. Flip and continue cooking on the other side. If the potatoes stick a little, gently pry them up, ensuring the golden brown bottoms are attached and add more butter. Once golden brown on both sides, they are ready to be served!

POTATO SKIN STARS

3-5 raw russet potatoes, choose longer, skinnier shaped potatoes

2 Tbsp salted butter

2 Tbsp olive oil

1. Peel the potatoes and place them in a container filled with water. Use a mandoline to slice the potatoes into potato chip thinness (½ centimeter). Aim for the longest and widest slices possible. (You can do this with a chef's knife if you have excellent knife skills.) Then place them back into the water container. You will need 5-6 "petals" per potato patty, approximately 40-48 petals in total. Any broken or partial pieces will not work.

2. Melt the butter on a plate in the microwave. Add and swirl in the olive oil.

3. Working in batches, retrieve 5-6 potato petals and shake or squeeze off excess moisture. Drag each one through the butter-oil mixture and lay it on a dinner-sized plate, not touching each other.

4. Microwave for 2-3 minutes to soften the potatoes.

5. Cool the petals for a minute. Lift and drip the butter-oil mixture back onto the plate.

6. Place the first petal on your work surface, perpendicular to yourself. Place the second petal on top of the first, but with the top point offset to the right. Adjust it so the bottom points are touching, and it is at about a 60-degree angle from the bottom. Place the third petal so it is touching the shared point of the other two, but the right side at an upward angle. Repeat until you have 5-6 petals in a circle with the base points overlapping and the rest spread out like the petals of a flower.

7. Place the potato patty in the center of the circle. Working from the last petal you laid down to the first, curl the petal over the patty, and repeat for all petals. They will meet in the center. Gently flatten the patty with your hand to fill any open pockets.

8. Repeat from step three until all the patties are enveloped in the petals.

9. Cook the stars as described in 'Cook the Tarts' or place in the fridge until needed.

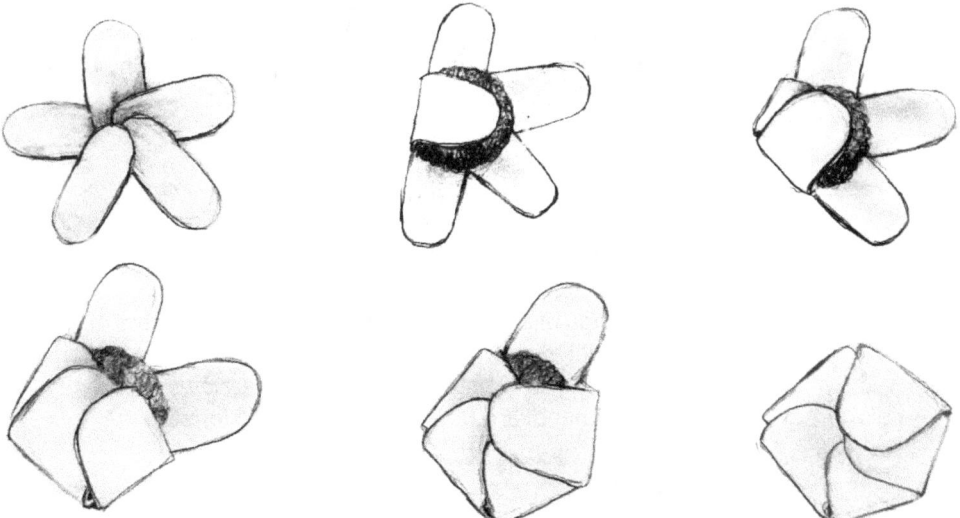

ILLUSTRATED BY: BENJAMIN ZABAN-BOYLAN *(LINE COOK)*   SMALL PLATES, SAUCES, & SIDES **114**

arroz verde

AVERY CASSAR 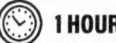 **1 HOUR** **SERVES 4-6 (1 CUP PORTIONS)**   **GLUTEN-FREE**   **VEGAN**   **DAIRY-FREE**

This recipe may seem unusual to Minnesota cooks, but it highlights a common way they prepare rice south of the border. The method of "frying" rice until it browns adds a toasted complexity to the finished product. You can substitute this recipe's greens with fresh herbs, an aromatic vegetable puree, or your favorite spice blends to create any flavor profile. We make Golden Rice 97 for our Paella with this method using dried spices in place of the pureed greens. Rice is rarely the star of any meal; however, it does not need to be a bland background.

gather

chef knife, paring knife, cutting board, measuring spoons, measuring cups, rondeau or heavy-bottomed medium-sized pot with lid, food processor or blender, long-handled spoon or rubber spatula

3 leaves kale, chopped

2 cloves garlic, chopped

1 fresh jalapeño, chopped

3 green onions, chopped

1 Tbsp parsley, de-stemmed

1 cup cilantro, de-stemmed

3 ½ cups water

¼ cup canola oil

1 ½ cups white basmati rice

1 ½ tsp kosher salt

1. As you prep each of the following ingredients, place them into a kitchen blender. Remove the stems from the kale and rough chop. De-seed and rough chop the jalapeño. Peel the garlic cloves. Rough chop the green onion and garlic.

2. De-stem the parsley and cilantro, then measure. Add 1 cup of water to the blender. Blend until pureed.

3. Heat a rondeau or medium-sized pot on high heat and add the canola oil. Wait one minute, then add the rice. Fry while stirring for 2-3 minutes until the kernels of rice become transparent.

4. Add the contents of the blender, but be careful of the steam. Add the salt, stir and let cook for about 5 minutes. The greens will need some time to steam.

5. When the sharp raw smell of garlic and onions turns to sweet softness, add the remaining 2 ½ cups of water. Boil, then lower the heat. Simmer until the water is down to the level of the rice.

6. Cover and turn the heat to the lowest setting. Set a timer for 5 minutes, then turn off the heat. Allow the steam to finish the rice. After about 10 minutes, open the lid and stir the rice to ensure even cooking. If there are crunchy pieces, re-cover and let sit for an additional 10-20 minutes.

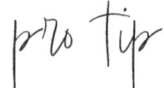

pro tip

Use the tongs of a fork to pull the leaves off the stems of parsley. This trick doesn't work with soft cilantro leaves, which is OK because cilantro stems taste good. Parsley stems, on the other hand, are bitter and best saved for stocks.

pimento cheese spread

JEREMY BARANY **25 MINUTES** **SERVES 8 (¼ CUP PORTIONS)**   **GLUTEN-FREE**   **VEGETARIAN**

If you head directly to the cheese platter at a party, this recipe is for you! Pimento Cheese is thick and creamy and, admittedly, an indulgence of mine. Try it on homemade crostinis or crackers. Bring Pimento Cheese to a potluck, but be prepared to come home with an empty bowl!

gather

measuring spoons, chef knife, microwave-safe bowl, food processor or blender, cheese grater, 16oz mason jar or serving container

¼ cup cream cheese

3 Tbsp mayonnaise
(Hellman's)

1 Tbsp + 1 ½ tsp sambal

⅛ tsp ground white pepper

¼ tsp smoked paprika

1 Tbsp minced jalapeño
(approx. ¼ jalapeño)

1 ¼ cup shredded cheddar

1 ¼ cup shredded aged white cheddar

2 Tbsp heavy cream

½ cup roasted red peppers, canned

1. Puree the first 8 ingredients in a food processor. A blender is more fussy, but works.

2. Warm the heavy cream in the microwave for 20 seconds, then pour it into the processor while it is running. Once fully combined, transfer the cheese mixture to a mixing bowl.

3. Strain the red peppers from the juice and gently squeeze out excess liquid, remove any stem and seeds. Mince, then fold into the cheese sauce. Taste test. If you would like a spicier spread, fold in more minced jalapeño or sambal.

4. Place the Pimento Cheese into one 16-ounce mason jar, or a serving dish, and chill for 2 hours.

It was a slamming busy day, and I was hosting. In my spare moments, I was helping my friends by watering the tables. At one point I looked up from the computer and said "Is that freaking Al Franken walking out the door right now?!" AJ, who had been his server, said "Yeah, you filled his water glass twice" I would have at least liked to smile at him!
- Melissa Weisser (server)

cranberry-peach chutney

**JACKIE FONTAINE
& JILLIAN FORTE**   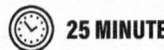 **25 MINUTES**   **SERVES 12 (⅓ CUP PORTIONS)**   **GLUTEN-FREE**   **VEGAN**   **DAIRY-FREE**

Prep cook Jackie and I created this recipe to preserve, and serve, an overabundance of ripe Georgia peaches. After a beautiful back-and-forth collaboration, we crafted a chutney with cranberries and tarragon. Originally, we paired the chutney with pecan and fresh herb-encrusted chicken breast and served it on a baguette with brie cheese as a sandwich special. It was so popular we put it on the menu. You can use this sweet peach chutney as a flavor-packed side to any dish. Try it on French Toast 38, with warm brie, on crackers, or even over vanilla ice cream!

gather

chef's knife, cutting board, heavy-bottomed pot, measuring cups, measuring spoons, scale, rubber spatula or wooden spoon, baking sheet

**1 medium shallot,
minced**

1 ½ cups cranberries,
fresh or frozen

**4 Tbsp +2 tsp white
sugar**

½ tsp kosher salt

2 Tbsp cider vinegar

2 lbs peaches, fresh or
frozen, 1-inch dice

**1 Tbsp fresh minced
tarragon**

1. Mince the shallot and place in a medium or large sauce pot. Add the cranberries, sugar, salt, and vinegar.

2. Turn the heat to medium and cook until the cranberries have popped and the mixture has the consistency of jam. You may need to squish the cranberries against the side of the pan with a wooden spoon. Add a dash of water if it looks dry.

3. Dice the peaches into approx. 1-inch cubes. If using fresh, cut around the pit, starting at the stem, then twist the flesh with the palms of your hands to separate the halves. Pull out the pit, slice the flesh into wedges, then 1-inch pieces. An under-ripe peach will keep the pit, making it hard to remove. In that case, cut the pit out.

4. Add the peaches to the cranberry paste in the pan and stir. Cook for about 15 minutes or until the peaches are soft. Do not cook them into mush. Stir occasionally, watching so the sugars don't scorch. If the pan starts to blacken, turn off the heat and allow the moisture to deglaze the pan.

5. De-stem the tarragon, mince and set aside.

6. Once the peaches are fork-able soft, pour the mix onto a baking sheet to cool. Sprinkle the tarragon on top and place it in the fridge to cool.

7. Mix the tarragon into the chutney. Pack into two 16-ounce glass mason jars for storage. It will keep for 3-4 weeks in the fridge.

award-winning rhubarb chutney

COLLEEN BETTS **1 HOUR** **SERVES 6 (⅓ CUP PORTIONS)**   **GLUTEN-FREE**   **VEGAN**   **DAIRY-FREE**

Colleen, who worked as a line cook, baker, and head chef during her time at the Cafe, entered this chutney creation in the annual Churches United in Ministry (CHUM) Rhubarb Festival contest. This tangy, sweet chutney won the Grand Prize! "I got nervous when the judges started coming down the tasting line." She said. "The first judge was [local kitchen maven] Bea Ojakangas!" Colleen still has the Rhubarb Festival t-shirt that was her "trophy."

gather

chef knife, cutting board, mixing bowl, baking sheet, rondeau, or heavy-bottomed pot

2 lbs rhubarb, fresh or frozen (approx. 8 stalks)

1 Tbsp canola oil, divided

1 tsp kosher salt

½ tsp black pepper

2 tsp minced shallot

2 tsp fresh minced ginger

1 tsp garam masala

¼ cup maple syrup

1 tsp minced red Fresno pepper or ½ tsp red pepper flakes

¼ cup craisins

¼ cup cider vinegar

1 tsp red pepper flakes

1. Heat the oven to 350°.

2. Cut rhubarb into 1-inch chunks and place in a mixing bowl. Pour 1-2 teaspoons canola oil over it, and sprinkle with salt and pepper. Mix and pour onto a greased baking sheet.

3. Bake for 20-25 minutes. This will soften and bring out the sweetness of the rhubarb. At the fifteen-minute mark, heat a heavy-bottomed rondeau on medium-low heat. Add 1-2 teaspoons canola oil and the shallots. Slowly sweat them for 2-3 minutes. Do not brown.

4. Add the ginger and continue to cook for an additional 3 minutes.

5. Add the garam masala and cook for 2 minutes.

6. Add all the remaining ingredients, including the rhubarb. Mix and cook on low heat for 10 minutes. Stir frequently. Note: Cooked sugars can easily scorch and give the dish a "caramelized" flavor. So keep the heat low. If you see brown or black spots on the pan, lower the heat, and use the spoon to rub the chutney over those spots and pull off the sugars. Also, be careful not to burn your fingers or tongue while tasting.

7. Allow the chutney to cool before putting it in a mason jar and covering it with a lid. Remember to label and date!

pro tip
Buy organic ginger root on sale and freeze the chunks: use a micro-plane zester to add "ginger snow" to anything: stir-fry, smoothies, pancakes, water bottle. -Colleen Betts (chef)

smoked salmon seasoning

AVERY CASSAR   **5 MINUTES**   **SERVES 8-10 (3 OZ PORTIONS)**   **GLUTEN-FREE**   **DAIRY-FREE**

Entire books and blogs have been written, and careers built, on the art of smoking meats. Rightfully so. Smoking is a time-honored, magnificent way to preserve and flavor all kinds of foods! Still, it seems a laborious process that only the dedicated can accomplish. Like butchering, the process is cloaked in mystique. Only the male chefs I'd worked with took on the task, and no one offered to teach me. Of course, to a plucky female chef, this meant the challenge was set! If I was ever to be an equal, I had to be proficient at these skills. So I put on my big girl pants, set aside my fear of failure, and boldly asked to be included. While learning to smoke salmon, I have overcooked, undercooked, and burned the fish. I've gotten it perfectly tender and covered it in soot. The worst was the time I started the parking lot on fire! (The spot is still visible by the smoker.) But, in truth, smoking is not that difficult, and you can transform mistakes into other delicious dishes; fish cakes, and "smokey" salmon chowder (occasionally given away as kitty food). Here are basic instructions for smoking fish, but if you find yourself intrigued, I suggest buying a book specific to your equipment or devoted to the topic. But try it. Think of me as your virtual cheerleader! You can do it!

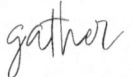 **spice or coffee grinder, measuring spoons, small mixing bowl, fish tweezers, maple wood, bucket of water, smoker, charcoal, newspaper, matches, metal spatula**

SALMON SEASONING

2 Tbsp whole coriander seeds

2 Tbsp whole fennel seeds

2 Tbsp whole black peppercorns

2 Tbsp kosher salt

6 Tbsp white sugar

3-4 lbs salmon

1. Grind the coriander, fennel, and peppercorns in a spice grinder or clean coffee grinder Pour into a small mixing bowl. Add the salt and sugar, and mix together.

"Never have I worked at a place where you put tips in an accordion folder after wrapping them in paper with staples and write 'I love you, here's your tip.'" - Faith Woodruff

PREPARING THE SALMON

1. Remove all the pin bones with fish tweezers or needle-nose pliers. Gently pull each one out at a low angle towards the head of the fish. Practice makes perfect!

2. Cut the salmon to your preferred serving size and place it on a sheet pan or in a baking dish. Heavily sprinkle the seasoning mix over the fish. Try to coat the sides as much as possible. The seasoning recipe will cover 3-4 lbs of salmon.

3. Let the fish sit uncovered in the fridge for 24 hours. The fish is going to release moisture, so do not put it at an angle or above ready-to-eat produce. Cross-contamination is dangerous.

SMOKED SALMON

A VERY BASIC GUIDE

1. Soak 1-2 pieces of maple wood in a bucket of water.

2. Prepare the charcoal chimney by filling the lower chamber with black and white newspaper or paper from the charcoal bag. Fill the upper chamber with charcoal. Light the paper and allow it to light the charcoal. Once the charcoal is glowing red, carefully pour it into the smoke box.

3. Place the soaked wood on top of the coals and close the box.

4. Put the salmon on the grates in the smoker (I prefer to place the salmon in the smoker sooner than later, so I don't get a face full of smoke). Note: Place the fish near the middle of the grate, but slightly closer to the smoker box, where the heat is highest.

5. Close the lid. Adjust the air vents. You want the smoke to be drawn through the chamber. To start, open the air vent into the smoker and out the chimney halfway. Play with the vents until you get a steady stream of exiting smoke.

6. Cook time depends on the size of your smoker, how much charcoal you used, and the amount of fish that you are smoking. Generally, I check the fish after about 20 minutes, but it typically takes closer to 30 or 40 minutes. I sometimes have to rotate the fish or take the pieces closest to the smoker box out before the others. I have learned that if the fish looks well smoked, but is not fully cooked, it's best to remove it from the smoker and place it in a 300° oven for about 3 minutes. This can cause the fish to be drier, but it's better than having bitter-soot-covered fish

tofu and tempeh (t&t) marinade

JILLIAN FORTE **10 MINUTES** **SERVES 10-16 (½ CUP TOTAL)**   **GLUTEN-FREE**   **DAIRY-FREE**   **VEGETARIAN**   **KETO**

My good friend Aleasha once made a salad with mysterious, tasty, crumbled bits on top. I thought it was bacon, but I was a vegetarian at the time, which she was well aware of. It turned out to be marinated tempeh that she had crumbled and fried! I was immediately hooked on the crunchy, umami goodness. When first employed at the Cafe, I suggested we create a similar marinade to use with our tofu and tempeh. Thus our T&T marinade was born. The tofu for our Thai Curry, and the tempeh for our TLT (Tempeh, Lettuce, Tomato,) sandwich are marinated in this sauce.

gather

measuring cups, spoons, mixing bowl, whisk

½ cup g.f. tamari.

1 Tbsp sesame oil

1 Tbsp +1 ½ tsp rice wine vinegar

½ tsp onion powder

½ tsp cayenne powder

1 tsp garlic powder

½ tsp ground cumin

¼ tsp ground coriander

1. Pour the tamari, oil, and vinegar into a bowl.

2. Sprinkle the dried spices over the liquid. This prevents clumping.

3. Whisk together and pour into a seal-able container.

4. To use, drizzle a small amount over the tofu or tempeh, and gently toss to cover. Discard any leftovers in the bowl. Do not pour it back into the container.

pro tip

Remember tofu and tempeh can carry bacteria. Avoid cross-contamination by washing hands before and after preparation.

"One of my most favorite memories of the Cafe is our first table-to-farm dinner at Farmer Sara's farm, Birch Point Gardens. Jillian and Avery smoking all those chicken thighs and the squash blossoms! Then Dean and the bonfire and the contraband keg of Leinenkugel's Octoberfest (which we thought was totally legal!) That was the start of a lovely summer of table-to-farm dinners. Birch Point, Food Farm, and beyond." - Sarah Runholt-Farrell

kirsten's hard-boiled eggs

KIRSTEN AUNE **25 MINUTES** **SERVES 6 (2 EACH)**   **GLUTEN-FREE**   **DAIRY-FREE**   **VEGETARIAN**   **KETO**

Everyone has a method for hard boiling eggs. This one is foolproof! It was passed down from the Benedictine Sisters of Saint Scholastica to Kirsten Aune, a talented prep cook at the Cafe. "Many of the Sisters grew up on farms in Southern Minnesota, Wisconsin, and Iowa," Kirsten explained. "They brought their tested and true rural recipes with them."

gather

4-quart pot

12 eggs

2-3 quarts water

1. Place the eggs and water into a large pot. Turn the heat on high.

2. Once the water comes to a rapid boil, turn off the heat and cover.

3. Set a timer for 20 minutes.

4. Drain and run cold water over the eggs until they are cool to the touch.

5. You can store eggs for 1 week in or out of their shells.

pro tip

It is easiest to peel the eggs just after they have cooled, maybe even still a little warm on the inside. Also, I have found that cracking eggs on the wider base, not the pointed tip, reduces the annoying way the white peels off in chunks. Cracking the shell sends air around the egg, separating the skin from the white. The prep cooks at the Cafe also noticed that older eggs peel easier than fresh ones.

Working at the Cafe gave me the opportunity to try many different positions. Even if some didn't work out it wasn't burning a bridge, it was more like "That isn't for you." The lifelong friendships supported me throughout college. It's a living career there. It even helped me buy my house. - Amanda Clark (server & graphic designer)

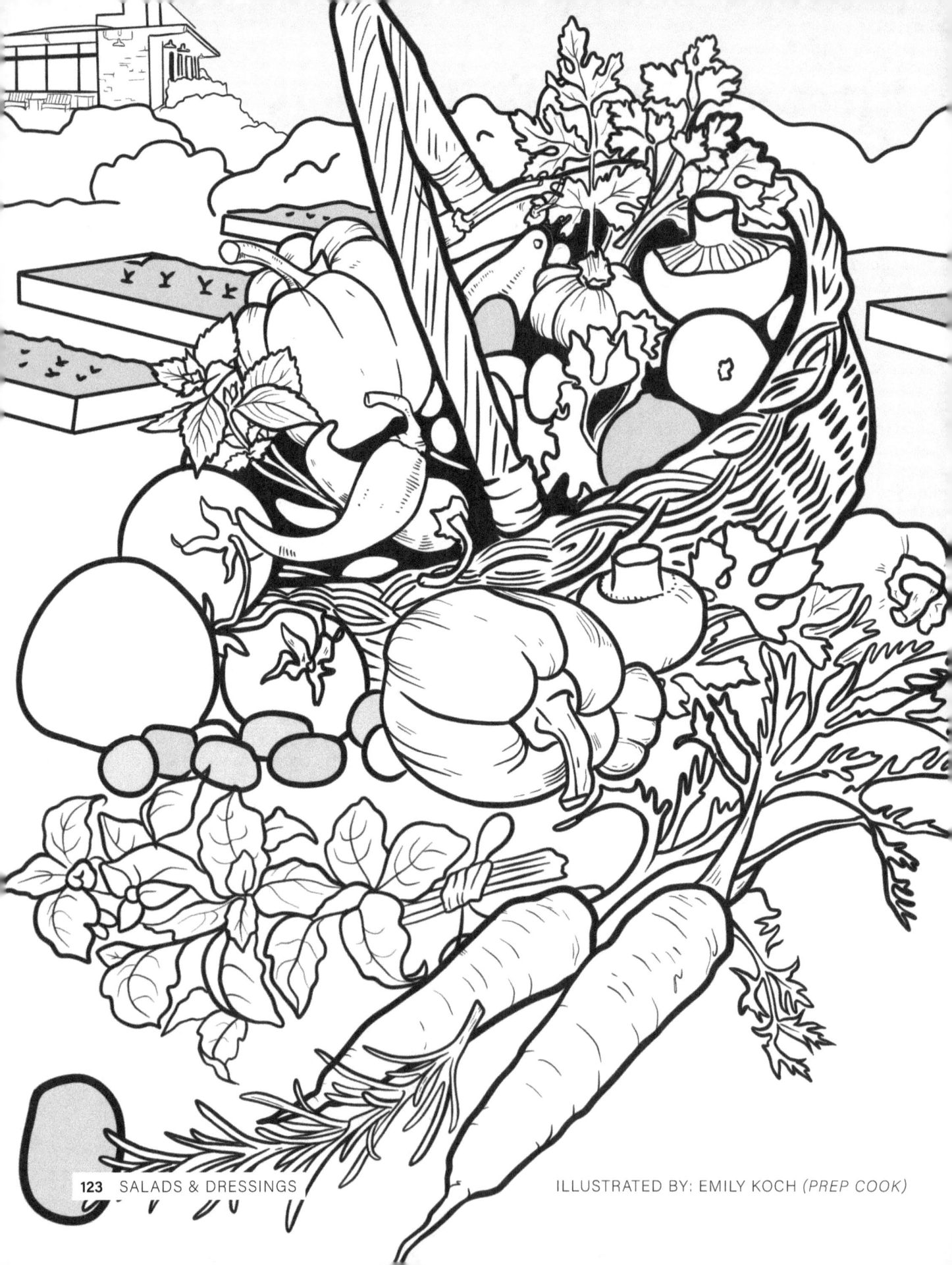

ILLUSTRATED BY: EMILY KOCH *(PREP COOK)*

salads & dressings

Salads are more than a healthy side dish, necessary but not necessarily joyful. A great salad is a truly lovely experience, each bite exploding with distinct flavors. At Sara's Table Chester Creek Cafe excels at creating salads for each season, a delight, particularly when our on-site gardens are flourishing. As a chef, strolling through the garden inspires my creativity— the taste of a warm tomato, the crunch of a haricot vert, and the colors and peppery flavor of the nasturtium blossoms— and allows my mind to ponder preparations. Crafting a salad with seasonal vegetables is exciting. Spinning up a vinaigrette that ties them together is food play at its finest.

The offerings in this section of the cookbook highlight the seasonal produce of the Northland. The Grilled Steak, Asparagus & Mushroom Salad can be made with wild foraged mushrooms, ramps, and fiddlehead ferns. My favorite, the Massaged Kale Salad, will easily support any highly producing vegetable plant in your garden from tomatoes, to baby carrots, to edible flowers. The Root Vegetable Panzanella warm-up northern winters with maple syrup-coated hearty greens, and a rainbow of roasted vegetables. The breakfast salad is exceptional year-round! Well-made salads feed the eye with form and color, intrigue the taste buds, and offer a variety of textures. They leave us with an energized body, lightness of spirit, and a thankful heart.

grilled steak, asparagus & mushroom salad with malbec vinaigrette

HEATHER ERICKSON & JILLIAN FORTE

 40 MINUTES

 SERVES 4 (ENTRÉE SIZED PORTIONS)

*GLUTEN-FREE

Heather and I designed this salad to be all about spring. The season when the snow has finally melted, the grass is turning green, and our thoughts turn to grilling outdoors. Spring in the Northland is asparagus season, but also the time of fiddlehead ferns, so feel free to switch them out. Hunt the woods for ramps to substitute for the onions, and keep an eye out for the season's first edible mushrooms! If you're a gardener, your first greens might be ready to harvest. This salad recipe is as fresh, timely, and local as it gets!

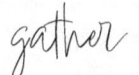 measuring spoons, measuring cups, mixing bowl, whisk, chef's knife, bread knife and cutting board, skewers, grill, tongs

MALBEC VINAIGRETTE

GLUTEN-FREE   ***DAIRY-FREE**   **VEGETARIAN**

½ cup Malbec wine or sweet red wine

1 Tbsp minced shallot or red onion

1 Tbsp + 1 ½ tsp white wine vinegar

¼ tsp kosher salt

1 pinch black pepper

¼ tsp white sugar

½ tsp honey

¼ cup extra virgin olive oil

¼ cup canola oil

1. Boil the Malbec wine and shallot in a small saucepan over medium-high heat. Reduce in half. Cool.

2. Place the vinegar, salt, pepper, sugar, and honey in a bowl. Add the wine and shallot mix. Whisk together as you slowly drizzle in the oils. Note: This vinaigrette does not contain a binder, such as mustard. It is going to separate. No worries, just give it a good stir before dressing the greens.

SALAD

4 4-6 oz hanger steaks
or your choice

1 tsp kosher salt

½ tsp black pepper

1 bunch asparagus

1 Tbsp canola oil

1 ½ cups crimini
mushrooms, halved
(approx. 1 container)

1 medium red onion,
quartered

1 loaf baguette or
French Bread

1 Tbsp salted butter

8 oz spring greens

¼ + cup gorgonzola or
Stilton *omit for d.f.

1. Light the grill.

2. Cut any silver skin or tough tendons from the hanger steak. Sprinkle the salt and pepper over the beef.

3. Snap the stems off the asparagus and set aside. Halve or quarter the mushrooms. Peel and quarter the onions. Cover both in olive oil and a pinch of salt. Skewer the mushrooms and onions in no particular order.

4. Slice 8 pieces of bread on a bias to get long, dramatic slices, then smear each with butter.

5. Grill the beef to your desired temp. (Although most chefs will tell you anything past medium-rare is overdone) See Pro Tip below. It's a good one.

6. Put the asparagus on a cooler side of the grill, tips facing the coolest part. Try not to burn those flavorful bits. The mushroom and onion skewers go on next, also not on the hottest side. Flip and grill everything until the asparagus is blistered and the mushrooms and onions are soft. Remove from the grill. Slide the mushrooms and onions off the skewer and set aside.

7. Toss the greens in ¼ cup Malbec Vinaigrette. Taste and add more if necessary. Divide and mound in the center of 4 plates. Fan out the asparagus and randomly scatter the mushrooms and onions on each plate.

8. Once the steak is done, pull it off the heat and let it rest for approx. 5 minutes.

9. Place the buttered bread slices on the grill, right where you cooked the steak. Watch carefully, this will not gently toast the bread but give it a charred meaty flavor while adding to its dramatic appearance with long black lines. Place two slices on each plate.

10. Slice the beef into ½-inch thick slices. Note: This is unnecessary; however, it is more elegant and you don't need to provide steak knives to everyone and watch them saw through their dinner. This also allows you to evenly divide the meat and check that it is done to your preference.

11. Layer the meat on the front of the plate, and crumble the blue cheese over the top. Another crack of fresh black pepper never hurt this salad!

pro tip

This was one of the first things I learned when working "grill side". It goes like this... Open and relax your hand, palm up, and now touch the fleshy part under your thumb. That spongy feeling is what a rare steak feels like when it's done cooking. Now just touch your thumb to your pointer finger and feel the fleshy spot again. It's a bit firmer, huh? That is a medium-rare steak. Middle finger touch (just lightly touching) is medium, the ring finger is medium-well and the pinky finger is well-done. *Also remember meat will continue to cook after you take it off the grill. It's better to under guess than over. You can cook it longer, but you can't take it back.

delicata, pickled beets & herbed goat cheese salad with mustard vinaigrette

JEREMY BARNAY **2 HOURS** **SERVES 4 ENTRÉES**   **VEGETARIAN**   **GLUTEN-FREE**   ***VEGAN**   ***DAIRY-FREE**

After I relinquished my position at the Cafe to follow my whims in Mexico, Jeremy Barnay, aka the Gentle Giant, created a host of tantalizing recipes. Though this salad requires a bit of prep time, it makes excellent use of fall harvest beets and squash. For this warm yet zippy salad, Jeremy chose sweet Delicata (delicate) squash. They are thin-skinned, thus spoil quickly, and often disappear from the stores around Christmas. If you can't find Delicata, Butternut is a great substitute. With their longer shelf-life, you can find them until March.

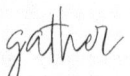 three medium-small pots, chef's knife, cutting board, liquid measuring cups & spoons, whisk, 3 mixing bowls, spoon, baking sheet & silicone mat or parchment paper, flat spatula, kitchen aid or blender, scale, tongs

PICKLED BEETS

4 medium red beets

1 cup cider vinegar

1 cup white wine vinegar

1 cup water

½ cup white sugar

1 ½ tsp kosher salt

1-2 allspice berries or ¼ tsp powder

1 clove or ¼ tsp ground

½ star anise

1. Boil a pot of water. Cut the tails and green stems off the beets. Place the beets in the water and boil until fork-able soft, approximately 45 minutes. Although it depends on their size.

   🔔 If making the whole dish, skip ahead to the Delicata.

2. Strain the water and cool the beets, just enough to work with them.

3. Combine the remaining ingredients in the same pot and bring to a simmer.

4. Peel and slice the beets into ½ -inch wide circles. Turn the heat off the brine and submerge the beets. Allow the liquid to cool without a lid in the fridge. Note: You can store pickled beets in the fridge for 2-3 weeks.

HERBED GOAT CHEESE

4-6 oz goat cheese (cheve) *vegan soft cheese

1 Tbsp fresh minced herbs (chive, dill, and parsley or 2 or more of any type)

1. Crumble the goat cheese (or vegan cheese) into a small mixing bowl

2. Mince the herbs together and add to the bowl. Extra herbs can be added to the cheese or sprinkled on the salad.

3. Mix with a fork if it's dry and crumbly or a rubber spatula if it is a wetter variety of chevre.

ROASTED DELICATA SQUASH & TOASTED PECANS

1 large Delicata squash or ½ Butternut

1 Tbsp canola oil

¼ cup maple syrup

1 tsp kosher salt

¼ tsp black pepper

¼ cup pecans, toasted

1. Heat the oven to 450°. If you have a convection option, use it for a crispier delicata.

2. Rinse and scrub the delicata to remove any soil. Cut off the stem and tail and slice lengthwise down the middle. Use a spoon to scrape out the seeds and discard them. Leave the edible and delicious skins on the squash. Lay each half flesh side down and cut ½ -inch slices or half-moons. Place in a mixing bowl.

3. Drizzle the canola oil and maple syrup over the slices. Sprinkle in the salt and pepper, and toss to combine. Place the squash slices, in a single layer, on a well-oiled or lined baking sheet. Pour any remaining liquid in the bowl over the squash.

4. Bake for 12 minutes in a conventional oven or 8 minutes on a convection setting or until the flesh is completely soft. Set aside and let cool.

    If making the whole dish, toast the raw pecans at the same time as the Delicata. They have a similar baking time. Place the nuts on a baking sheet and place them in the oven, below the squash. Stir once at the 6-minute mark.

MUSTARD VINAIGRETTE

¾ tsp kosher salt

¼ tsp black pepper

1 Tbsp minced shallot

2 Tbsp whole grain mustard

1 Tbsp dijon mustard

2 ½ tsp honey *sub agave or maple syrup

¼ cup cider vinegar

½ cup extra virgin olive oil

¼ cup canola oil

1. Combine the salt, pepper, minced shallot, whole grain & dijon mustard, honey, and cider vinegar into a food processor or mixing bowl.

2. Turn on the food processor and slowly drizzle in the oils until fully emulsified. Alternately, whisk the first ingredients together in a mixing bowl. Slowly drizzle in the oil. Taste, adjust, then set aside.

SALAD

8 oz hearty greens mix (spinach, arugula, kale, romaine)

1. Put the salad greens into a mixing bowl and pour ¼ cup of the vinaigrette over them. Use tongs to mix. Taste a leaf to ensure there is enough vinaigrette as it's easier to start with less and add more. Pile the greens onto 4 dinner-sized plates.

2. Crumble or dollop the chevre cheese onto each pile of greens. Be generous with the cheese as it is the primary fat and lends a beautiful creaminess to the dish.

3. Lay alternating beet and delicata slices around the rim of the salad. Sprinkle with toasted pecans.

asparagus & poached egg salad with lemon-dijon vinaigrette

AVERY CASSAR 🕐 **40 MINUTES** 👥 **SERVES 2** ***VEGETARIAN** ***GLUTEN-FREE** ***DAIRY-FREE**

I have tasted many salads during my 16 years at the Cafe, but this one of Avery's is truly memorable for its elegance. Parts of the preparation are challenging, like shaving the asparagus and making pancetta rounds, but you'll find that the salad is much sexier with the smooth, almost creamy, asparagus curls and the bright red, flavor-forward wheels. It's not hard to imagine this salad being served at a Parisian sidewalk cafe, but the lake view from our patio at the Cafe is superior.

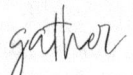 **gather** **mixing bowl, whisk, cast iron pan, small sauce pot, peeler, bread knife, chef knife, measuring spoons**

LEMON-DIJON VINAIGRETTE

½ tsp fresh minced tarragon or basil

½ tsp kosher salt

¾ tsp dijon

1 tsp honey

1 ½ tsp cider vinegar

1 ½ tsp lemon juice

¼ tsp lemon zest

1 Tbsp extra virgin olive oil

1 ½ tsp canola oil

1. Mince the tarragon and place it in a small bowl. Add the salt, dijon, honey, and cider vinegar.

2. Zest ¼ of the lemon into the bowl. Juice half the lemon into a separate bowl. Measure it and add it to the bowl with the other ingredients.

3. Whisk everything together. Slowly pour in both oils. Taste and adjust to your preference.

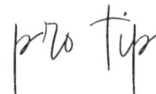 **pro tip**

Mustard is the secret ingredient to making a vinaigrette emulsify or bind. It helps the oil and vinegar, which notoriously do not bond together, create a consistent salad dressing. Add as little as a ½ teaspoon of either dried or prepared mustard to any vinaigrette.

SALAD

1 Tbsp white vinegar

8 pre-sliced pancetta rounds

½ loaf baguette or French Bread

4 eggs

12-16 spears asparagus

4-6 oz arugula

2 oz pea shoots (optional)

4 oz Parmesan wedge or shredded *omit for d.f.

1. Simmer 2 quarts of water, then add 1 tablespoon of white vinegar.

2. Place as many slices of pancetta as will fit without overlapping in a cold cast iron pan. Try to keep their round shape. Turn the heat to medium and brown the pancetta until crisp, flipping as needed. Repeat until all rounds are cooked. Place them on a paper towel to remove excess fat.

   🔔 While waiting for the wheels to cook, poach the eggs).

3. Poach one egg at a time. Pull the egg out of the water, using a slotted spoon, and place it in a bowl while the others are cooking. See Poached Eggs below for pointers. If poaching eggs seems like too much work or you are short on time, soft-boil the eggs. Place them in the pot of boiling water and simmer for 5-6 minutes. Cool, then peel.

4. Cut the bread on a long bias. Once the pancetta is done, pour a teaspoon of olive oil into the cast iron and gently toast the bread. Turn off the heat and let it stay in the pan as a warming spot.

5. Shave the asparagus. Hold the tough stem in one hand. Place the asparagus on the cutting board, with the stem in your hand hanging off the edge. Using a peeler, start at the point where the asparagus is turning from white to green, then shave away from yourself. Rotate the spear until it's a nub, toss the fibrous stem, and repeat with each stalk. It's easier than it sounds; however, you can always snap off the fibrous section and then cut the tender part into long thin strips.

6. Dress the arugula, shaved asparagus, and pea shoots with 2 tablespoons of Lemon-Dijon vinaigrette. Taste and add more dressing if needed. Divide the greens onto two plates.

7. Sprinkle or shave the Parmesan onto each salad. Set two poached eggs in the center of each pile of greens. Take the 4 nicest-looking pancetta wheels and place two on each salad. In a small bowl, use your hands to crumble the remaining pancetta pieces as finely as possible. Sprinkle the salads with the pancetta "dust". Lean 2 pieces of toast on the eggs.

POACHED EGGS

Simmer a small pot of water, just a few bubbles, and add 1 tablespoon of white distilled vinegar. Using a large spoon, gently stir the water on the outside edge of the pot, creating a "hurricane effect" but not too fast, more slowly. Crack one egg directly into the center. The swirling water should wrap the tendrils of the egg whites into the center, creating a tight, uniform shape. Now, wait for about 5 minutes before gently scooping the egg out with a slotted spoon. If you have ever watched the movie, *Julie and Julia*, you may know how difficult but ultimately rewarding a perfectly poached egg can be.

root vegetable panzanella with maple-sherry vinaigrette

**BRUCE WALLIS &
PETER RAVINSKI** **1 HOUR & 30 MINUTES** **SERVES 4** *GLUTEN-FREE *VEGETARIAN *VEGAN *DAIRY-FREE

Minnesotans are all keenly aware of how freaking cold it gets in winter. There are days when we just want to snuggle in and eat heavy foods. Yet after a while, we know we should eat a meal that is a bit more, well... healthy. This salad strikes the perfect balance of health and comfort food. It's best when the veggies are right out of the oven, and the homemade croutons are crispy chunks. The hearty greens are tossed in a sweet maple-sherry vinaigrette and sprinkled with savory Parmesan peels. Not comforted enough? Add a baked chicken breast.

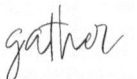 **chef's knife, cutting board, aluminum foil, serrated knife, 2-3 mixing bowls, 2 baking sheets, vegetable peeler, spatula, paring knife, measuring spoons and cups, whisk, mixing spoon**

CROUTONS

¼ loaf un-sliced bread (approx. 4 inches)
*sub g.f. bread

1 ½ tsp kosher salt

½ tsp garlic powder

¼ tsp powdered oregano or thyme
(optional)

¼ tsp onion powder
(optional)

🔔 If making the whole dish, start with the Roasted Root Vegetables.

1. Cut the bread into 1-inch cubes. Place in a mixing bowl. Drizzle with 1 teaspoon olive oil. Sprinkle with a pinch of salt and ¼ teaspoon garlic powder, and half of the optional spices. Toss or mix. Add another teaspoon of oil, a pinch of salt and ¼ teaspoon garlic powder, and the other half of the additional spices. Toss together. Place on a baking sheet. See Recipe Tip below.

2. Bake the croutons for 10 minutes.

   🔔 If making the whole dish, wait until the root vegetable timer goes off. If adding a chicken breast to the salad, place it on the crouton pan, but off to one side, not touching the croutons.

3. When the timer dings, pull the croutons out of the oven. Give them a stir. Usually, the ones on the perimeter are crispy and the ones in the center are soft. Continue baking for 5-10 minutes.

4. Check the croutons. They are ready when the outside is crispy. A soft center is great for immediate eating, but if you plan to serve the salad later, they need to be crunchy all the way through to the inside (cold, soft croutons seem stale).

recipe tip: Good croutons are those with a fair bit of oil, more seasoning than you think, and not too much salt! You can always pop an uncooked crouton into your mouth to check if it's good. -Christopher Sheppard (prep cook)

ROASTED ROOT VEGETABLES

3 small beets

3 Tbsp canola oil

2 medium parsnips,
1-inch dice

**1 sweet potato or yam or
2 carrots,** 1-inch dice

½ rutabaga, 1-inch dice

1 tsp kosher salt

1. Heat the oven to 425°. Lightly grease a baking sheet.

2. Cut the tail and greens off the beets and rinse off any soil. Place in the middle of a sheet of aluminum foil. Drizzle with 1 teaspoon canola oil, then wrap in the foil. Place the foil packet in the oven. Set a timer for 20 minutes.

   🔔 At that point, you will put the next batch of veggies in the oven. However, the beets will stay in the oven for over an hour, so let them cook while all the action is happening.

3. Peel and cut the parsnips into 1-inch pieces. Place them in a mixing bowl and drizzle a little canola oil over them. Add a pinch of salt and toss together. Lay them on the greased baking sheet, off to one side. Repeat with the sweet potato or yam and rutabaga, ensuring each vegetable is separate. Note: Keeping root vegetables apart on the baking sheet prevents over or under baking the vegetables. When one veggie is done, you can easily remove it from the pan while allowing the others to continue cooking.

4. When the 20-minute timer goes off (from the beets), put the root veggies in the oven. Add another 20 minutes to the timer.

   🔔 If making the whole salad, start on the croutons and dressing.

5. Rotate the pan in the oven and set the timer for 10 minutes.

   🔔 If making the whole salad, put croutons in the oven now.

6. When the timer goes off, pull the veggies out of the oven. Fork test each of the vegetables for softness. If one or more is not soft, remove the finished veggies with a spatula and place them in a mixing bowl. Return the unfinished veggies to the oven and set a 5-minute timer. As each vegetable finishes, put it in the mixing bowl.

7. Test a beet. They are done when a paring knife easily slides into the center of the beet. Cool in the fridge, still wrapped in foil (this will aid in the skins peeling off easily).

8. Peel and cut the beets into 1-inch cubes. Add to the bowl with the other root vegetables and mix.

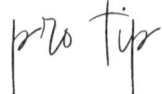

pro tip

Keep the oven door shut. Every second you leave the oven door open, you lose two degrees of heat. Thus, leaving it open for even 10 seconds will drop the temp by 20 degrees! It takes an oven time to warm back up again, making the cooking time longer. It's better to pull something out of the oven, close the door, test it, then return it rather than holding the door open.

MAPLE-SHERRY VINAIGRETTE

1 ½ tsp minced shallot or red onion

1 tsp dijon mustard

1 ½ tsp maple syrup

2 Tbsp sherry vinegar or red wine vinegar

6 Tbsp canola oil

2 Tbsp extra virgin olive oil

1. Finely mince the shallot and place it in a mixing bowl. Add the mustard, maple syrup, and vinegar. Whisk together.

2. Slowly drizzle in the oils while continuing to whisk until emulsified.

SALAD

¼ cup pecans, toasted

6-8 oz hearty salad greens mix (spinach, chard, kale, romaine)

4 oz Parmesan wedge or shredded *sub vegan cheese or omit

1. If you haven't already, put the pecans on a baking sheet and place them in the oven for 7 minutes or until fragrant. Set aside to cool.

2. Dress the greens with 2-3 tablespoons of the vinaigrette. Taste and add more vinaigrette if needed.

3. Pour 1-2 tablespoons of the vinaigrette over the Roasted Root Vegetables and stir.

4. Put the dressed greens into the same bowl as the root vegetables, add the croutons, and mix. Divide onto 4 large salad plates. Shave Parmesan on top of each salad with a vegetable peeler. Sprinkle with the toasted pecans.

"The best thing that Barb ever did was give me that little dog named Mandy. She adopted a white poodle dog down in Texas and brought it home. She was going to be leaving again for another trip, so she asked me if I could take care of the dog. I said sure. And when they came (back), she said just to keep the dog. I did and... I really bonded with (Mandy). I loved that dog." Diane Bailey

Barb would bend over backward for people. She really believed in micro-loans and would give them to staff, myself included, and then take it out of paychecks. They bought those houses and let people live in them, paid for lawyers at least once, and bailed people out of jail. I think of the time when Ella/Erin was born. Barb handed me a personal check for $500, unprompted when I was going to Florida, just "You're going on vacation, here, have some fun," she said. I didn't even see it coming, just a heart of gold, really. There were times when she gave me a raise. "You seem like you're having trouble. How much more do you need?" I have gotten married, had three children, and bought two houses while working here. I couldn't have done it without Barb.
- Peter Ravinski (operations manager)

"I became the bathroom maven, and I was until the day I left. I was going to calculate how many toilets I have cleaned over the 15 years of work. All 4, 5 days a week for 15 years. I had my special cleaner, 7th Generation. If I'm going to do it, I'm not going to use weird chemicals."
Sonja Helland (server) (Sonja cleaned around 15,600 toilets!!!)

spinach, feta & tomato breakfast salad with goddess dressing

HEATHER ERICKSON 35 MINUTES SERVES 4   GLUTEN-FREE   *VEGETARIAN   *VEGAN   *KETO

Salad for breakfast may be a foreign concept for many. Think of the greens as a bread replacement. This recipe showcases crispy bacon, creamy avocado, briny feta, and bright tomatoes. I like to add a hard-boiled egg for extra protein. Vegetarians simply need to switch the bacon for T&T Marinated tempeh 121. The accompanying Goddess Dressing is versatile. Make it with mayonnaise and sour cream, or with Vegan Aioli 55.

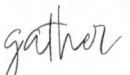 **blender or food processor, zester, mixing bowl, rubber spatula, sauté pan, paper towels, chef knife, cutting board, mixing bowl, whisk, measuring spoons, and cups**

GODDESS DRESSING

2 Tbsp mayonnaise
*sub Vegan Aioli 55

1 Tbsp sour cream
*sub Vegan Aioli 55

¼ ripe avocado

1 ½ tsp cider vinegar

½ tsp lemon juice

2 Tbsp minced green onion

1 Tbsp fresh minced parsley

1 Tbsp fresh minced chives

1 Tbsp fresh minced tarragon

⅛ tsp sea salt or kosher

⅛ tsp white sugar

1 Tbsp extra virgin olive oil

1. Place the mayonnaise, sour cream, avocado, vinegar, juice, and zest from ¼ of a lemon into a kitchen blender. Blend until the avocado has become completely creamy. Transfer to a mixing bowl.

2. Mince the green onion, parsley, chives, and tarragon. Add to the mixing bowl.

3. Add the salt and sugar to the bowl. Whisk together as you slowly pour in the olive oil. Taste the dressing and adjust it to your preference.

SALAD

8 slices bacon *sub tempeh strips + T&T Marinade 121

6-8 oz spinach

¾ avocado

1 pint cherry tomatoes, halved

½ cup feta crumbles

1. Cook the bacon or tempeh slices in the oven or stovetop. The stovetop is faster but can splatter. When crispy or browned, set on paper towels to dab up excess fat. Cut the strips into ½-inch pieces.

2. Slice the remaining ¾ avocado. See Avocado Tip 29.

3. Rinse and halve the cherry tomatoes. See Cherry Tomato Halves Tip 29.

4. Mix the spinach with 3-4 tablespoons of the dressing in a mixing bowl. It is a thick dressing, so spread it around until clump-free.

5. Place the greens on the plates, add the avocado slices, cherry tomatoes, bacon, or tempeh pieces, and sprinkle with the feta. Add a scrambled or hard-boiled egg for extra protein.

massaged kale salad

RITA B BERGSTEDT **25 MINUTES** **SERVES 6 (SIDE SIZED PORTIONS)**   **GLUTEN-FREE**   **VEGAN**   **DAIRY-FREE**

In my opinion, this salad is the absolute best way to eat kale. The kale is fresh, thus retaining its full nutritional value, while the massage makes it soft, tender, and lovely to eat. The combination of tamari and lime gives it a savory/tart flavor, and the fat from the avocado makes it creamy and smooth. This salad is my first choice for a quick vegetable side. It's amazing with Beef Bulgogi Tacos 70, Vietnamese Braised Beef Short Ribs 85, Green Buddha Bowl 83, over rice noodles, and on its own. The numerous mentions of it in this cookbook are proof of my undying love!

gather

chef's knife, cutting board, measuring spoons, mixing bowl

1 large bunch kale, rough chop (approx. ½ lb)

2 Tbsp canola oil

1 tsp sesame oil

1 Tbsp + 1 ½ tsp g.f. tamari or soy sauce

1 Tbsp lime juice

1 large carrot, shredded

1 whole avocado, optional

2 tsp sesame seeds, pre-toasted

1. De-stem the kale, then rough chop the leaves into approx. 1-2-inch squares. See Kale Tip 29. Place the kale into a mixing bowl, then pour the oils, tamari, and lime juice on top.

2. Massage the kale. What I really mean here is to squeeze the living daylights out of the kale. You will see the kale turn from a pale to dark green color as you break the cell walls, showing you have finished with the massage.

3. Peel the carrot or wash really well, then shred on a box grater. Scatter this on top of the kale. Dice the avocado and sprinkle it over the salad. See Avocado Tip 29. Note: The avocado will turn brown after a day in the fridge. If you won't be eating all the salad in the first sitting, just add avocado to the amount you will eat.

4. Sprinkle the sesame seeds on top and stir everything together with a wooden spoon, breaking apart any avocado pieces that are stuck together. Taste everything for a salty and zingy combo. Add more tamari or lime to adjust.

Thanks, Barb and Carla. You care about the employees and the environment, and that is really different from a lot of restaurants. It was the first restaurant that I knew to compost, and it was amazing.
- Faith Woodruff (FOH manager)

blue cheese dressing

JILLIAN FORTE **15 MINUTES** **SERVES 10-12 (1 ½ CUPS TOTAL)**   **VEGETARIAN**   **GLUTEN-FREE**

I love to smear creamy dressings all over my healthy greens. This recipe's fresh herbs blended with chunks of blue cheese are a delight. As is always the case with blues, choose a high-quality mature one like Stilton, or Gorgonzola.

gather

chef's knife, cutting board, blender or food processor, measuring cups, measuring spoons, rubber spatula

½ cup mayonnaise
(Hellmans)

¼ cup sour cream

¼ cup buttermilk

½ - ¾ cup blue cheese,
crumbled

½ tsp fresh minced garlic

½ tsp fresh minced parsley

¼ tsp fresh minced sage

¼ tsp fresh minced thyme

¼ tsp onion powder

¼ tsp kosher salt

¼ tsp black pepper

½ tsp red wine vinegar

1 dash Worcestershire sauce

1. Combine the mayonnaise, sour cream, buttermilk, and half of the blue cheese crumbles in a food processor or kitchen blender. Puree until smooth. Transfer to a mixing bowl.

2. Mince the garlic and fresh herbs. Add to the bowl.

3. Add the remaining half of the blue cheese, onion powder, salt, pepper, vinegar, and Worcestershire sauce. Mix with a rubber spatula.

I hated blue cheese for years! Yet I couldn't help but notice my coworkers sneaking bites of Stilton with guilty glee. I figured I should taste it, repeatedly. On the third try, my mind opened. I could taste the multiple levels of flavor: the tart, tangy, creamy, crunchy bits, and savoriness. It became a treasure to value. I am now a blue cheese snob. If you are new to blues and feel daunted by the blue cheese selection at your grocery store, look for a Stilton, Gorgonzola, or Roquefort. Skip the crap in a tub. - Jillian Forte

10,000 lakes dressing

JEREMY BARANY **15 MINUTES**  **SERVES 6-8 (1 CUP TOTAL)**   **GLUTEN-FREE**   **VEGETARIAN**   ***VEGAN**   **DAIRY-FREE**

This hopped-up version of 1,000 Island dressing may require a trip to the store, but its special ingredients are well worth the outing. It's the capers, cornichons (and Minnesota pride) that expand 1,000 islands to 10,000 lakes! Use this dressing on a Reuben sandwich, a hamburger, or a salad.

gather — **chef's knife & cutting board, measuring cups and spoons, food processor or mixing bowl, whisk**

2 Tbsp minced yellow onion

1 Tbsp cornichons or baby dill pickles

1 ½ tsp capers

½ cup mayonnaise *sub vegan aioli

2 ¼ tsp white sugar

⅛ tsp kosher salt

¼ tsp black pepper

2 Tbsp ketchup

1 ½ tsp white vinegar

1. Blend the onions, cornichons, and capers in a food processor into ⅛-inch pieces. Alternatively, mince them on the cutting board. Place in a mixing bowl.

2. Add the remaining ingredients to the bowl and whisk together. Taste and adjust to your preference.

My favorite story from filming Diners, Drive-In's & Dives was when I almost singed his famous hair. I removed a brisket from the oven, set it on the stovetop, then peeled off the foil and parchment paper cover and also set it on the stovetop. Quickly, a pilot light lit the parchment on fire. Not a big deal for a seasoned cook. I quickly grabbed the foil and folded it to smother the fire. As this was happening, the ashes from the paper began being sucked up by the hood system with a few pieces landing on Guy's gelled blond spiky hair. Suddenly someone yelled "The hair!!" and 5 people ran over to make sure his hair wasn't on fire. Oops.
- Jillian Forte

raspberry vinaigrette

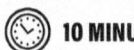 **10 MINUTES** 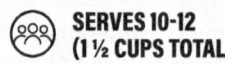 **SERVES 10-12 (1 ½ CUPS TOTAL)**   **GLUTEN-FREE**   **VEGETARIAN**   **VEGAN**   **DAIRY-FREE**

This is one of the Cafe's oldest recipes and a favorite for years. The raspberry jam we serve as a side is the base for this vinaigrette. Customers rave about our jam and want to either buy some or get the recipe to make at home. We always giggle because it's Smucker's. What can I say? In the business, a few items are better bought than made.

gather

food processor or bowl and whisk, measuring cups and spoons

¼ cup red wine vinegar

⅓ cup raspberry preserves (Smuckers)

½ tsp kosher salt

½ tsp black pepper

2 tsp lemon juice

1 ½ tsp orange juice

⅓ cup olive oil

⅓ cup canola oil

1. Combine the vinegar, raspberry preserves, salt and pepper, lemon, and orange juice in either a mixing bowl or food processor.

2. Whisk or blend together. While whisking, drizzle in the oils until they emulsify.

pro tip

The classic salad combination is fruit, cheese, and a nut. Think pears, bleu cheese and pecans or strawberries, Chevre and walnuts. If you choose berries as the fruit, try this dressing!

Chester Creek was my first "real job" at 16 years old, and in the beginning, I definitely acted like a 16-year-old. Growing up and waiting tables there for five years taught me a ton about food and being a good coworker. Most importantly, it let me hang out with some really amazing humans while on the clock. - Anders Jefferson (server)

One morning the opening line cook didn't show up to work, so the next person scheduled was called to come in ASAP. While quickly preparing the restaurant to open, the staff called the late person once more. Suddenly, they heard a ringing sound from the fireplace. Peering over the coffee bar, they found Peter V. sleeping on the old green couch! Turns out he had been out until late the night before and decided it would be easier to get to the Cafe at 3 am, take a nap on the couch, and then start work at 6! Half success.

The women frequently have clothing exchanges at the restaurant. We bring in our old clothes and let others take them for free. There is always wine and giggles while trying on clothes and getting new pieces. One time we held it in the dining room and piled the clothes on the booths and tables. At the end, we all cleaned up and went home with our treasures. The next morning, a customer called over their server, held up a piece of lacy clothing, and said "I think someone forgot.... something!!!"

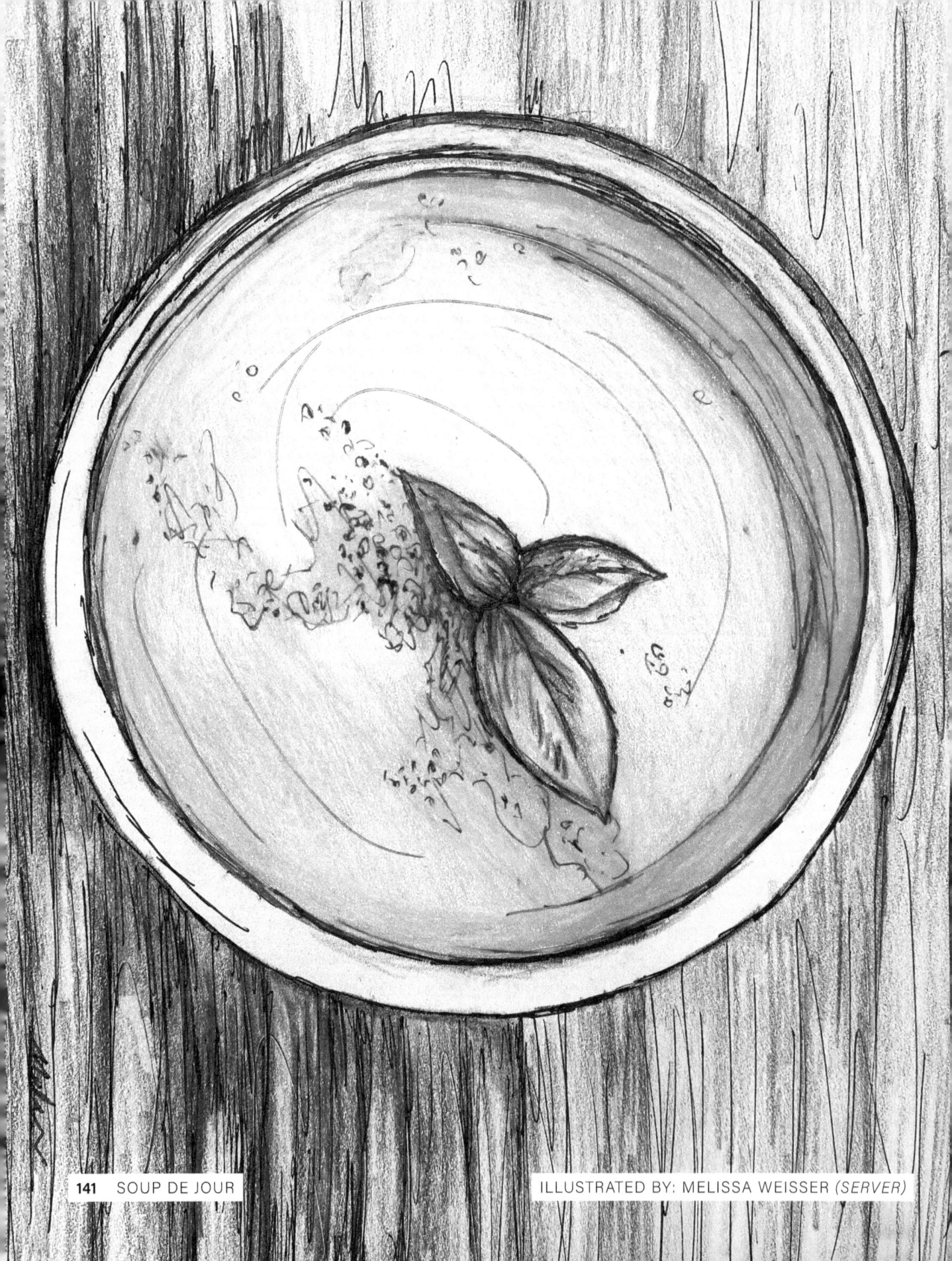

ILLUSTRATED BY: MELISSA WEISSER (*SERVER*)

soup de jour

Soup-making is an art born of tweaks, knowledge, and intuition. As is true with the practice of any art, skill increases with experience. Soup outcomes will vary based on the quality of your ingredients and your stock. Once your recipe is complete, taste a spoonful of the broth, close your eyes and evaluate the flavor profile. Does the soup seem flat or dull? Does it make your mouth water? Is it too salty? Not spicy enough? You can adjust the flavor if you understand what the soup needs. As always, start with small additions and gradually increase!

Try adding a little citrus to the Thai Chicken Coconut Soup. With its creamy base, it may need more acid or brightness. To enhance the umami of the Veggie Loaded Beef Stew, add tamari or Worcestershire. The Pork Pho Noodle Bowl often needs more fish sauce. Soups like the Ginger Carrot Quinoa and Curried Winter Squash should tease with their sweetness. An extra pinch of brown sugar, or a splash of maple syrup, may be what's called for. The Golden Gohbi Matar and Roasted Corn Poblano Chowder lend themselves well to added cayenne, or hot sauce. Soup pro, Heather Erickson says, "If you are still not satisfied with your soup's flavor, venture beyond the more obvious. Fresh herbs always make soup better." You can even try a drizzle of infused oil which will explode the flavors.

With practice and critical thinking, you can create memorable soups that leave your palate wanting more. Analyze your soups, experiment, and have fun playing with the flavors. When you sit down to eat, remember to stop judging and enjoy!

making stock

Making stock seems like a task only homesteaders or remote workers might take on. However, they are uncomplicated and basically made from simmering scraps. This list 'Great in Stocks' is only a guideline. Feel free to throw in any leftover vegetable bits you have, though keep in mind your final soup, or goal. I add squash seeds and apple cores when making the Curried Winter Squash Soup 154, but don't add them to the stock for Roasted Corn Poblano Chowder 155. It's important to remember to always include 2 parts onion, 1 part carrots, and 1 part celery (aka mirepoix) in every stock for that classic stock taste. Homemade stock will allow for control of the salt content and take your soup flavors to the next level.

GREAT IN STOCKS!

onion ends, some skins

leeks, whole or just green tops

celery, not too many leaves

fennel, save the fronds for garnish

carrot, tops and tips, some peelings

parsnip, tops, and tips

tomatoes, fresh, canned, or paste

broccoli stems

winter squash seeds

apple cores, 1-2 maximum

mushroom stems, or whole

garlic cloves

parsley stems or whole

fresh woody-stemmed herbs

bay leaves - always

peppercorns

OMIT FROM STOCKS

basil, cilantro and tarragon

potatoes, although a few peelings are OK

sweet potatoes

leafy greens

beets

cabbage

red onions

zucchini

green beans

cucumbers

pro tip

When prepping vegetables, keep a stock scrap bowl next to you. Transfer the scraps into a 1 gallon zip-top bag and freeze. Keep adding to the bag. When it's full, it's time to make a stock.

why not add these vegetables?

Many of the items on the Omit list can turn stock a strange color (red onions make purple stock and beets a deep red color), do not enhance the flavor, and can muddle the taste.

vegetable stock

PETER RAVINSKI **1 HOUR & 15 MINUTES** **MAKES 3+ QUARTS**   **GLUTEN-FREE**   **VEGAN**   **DAIRY-FREE**

This is so quick to make that you can pop it on the stove when you get home from work and it will be ready to pour into a soup an hour later. Hint: to avoid bitterness, don't simmer veggie stock longer than 2 hours.

gather

cutting, board, chef's knife, long handled spoon, stock pot, fine mesh strainer

2 cups onion scrap or pieces

1 cup carrot scraps or pieces

1 cup celery scrap or pieces

2-4 cups vegetable scraps, fresh or frozen

2-3 stems parsley and/ or thyme

4-6 cloves garlic

4-5 bay leaves

1 Tbsp black peppercorns

1 tsp kosher salt

1 gallon cold water

1. Place all the vegetable scraps, bay leaves, peppercorns, and salt into a stockpot. Add 1 gallon of cold water and bring to a boil. Note: If you want a richer flavor, sauté the vegetables first, deglaze with a splash of white wine, then add the remaining ingredients.

2. Lower heat and let simmer, covered, for 1 hour.

3. Strain through a fine-mesh strainer. Discard the pulpy veggies. Freeze any leftover stock. See Freezing Tip 30.

pro tip

Always use cold water for stock and soup making. Hot water has been sitting in a water heater for hours and often tastes metallic.

Sara's Table is one of a kind. I stumbled upon it, and it changed my life. I met some of my very best friends there, and working there helped me to realize my passion for sustainability and local farms. The support of coworkers and people I met while working at the Cafe helped me to do things I otherwise might not have done. - Anna Brown (bartender)

chicken stock

PETER RAVINSKI **4-8 HOURS** **MAKES 3+ QUARTS**   **GLUTEN-FREE**   **DAIRY-FREE**

The difference between chicken and vegetable stock is the addition of chicken bones and a longer simmer time. Only use raw chicken bones, never cooked. (Ask for bones from the butcher at your grocery store.) If you can't find raw bones, try a combination of cheap meat cuts, chicken wings, feet, and whatever you can find. We butcher whole chickens at the Cafe, allowing us to freeze bones and skin in preparation for stock-making day.

gather   **cutting, board, chef's knife, long handled spoon, stock pot, fine mesh strainer**

2 cups onion scrap or pieces

1 cup carrot scraps or pieces

1 cup celery scrap or pieces

2-3 cups vegetable scraps, fresh or frozen

4-5 bay leaves

2-4 stems parsley and/ or thyme

1 Tbsp black peppercorns

1 tsp kosher salt

2-4 lbs chicken bones

1 gallon cold water

1. Put vegetable scraps, bay leaves, peppercorns, and salt into a stockpot. Add 1 gallon of cold water. Put the raw chicken bones into the pot, then bring to a gentle simmer.

2. If possible, place the stock pot half on the burner and half off. This creates a circular motion in the pot and pushes any impurities off to the side, which you can easily scoop out and discard.

3. Simmer uncovered or partially covered for 4-6 hours. Do not let the stock boil. Boiling will emulsify the chicken fat, leaving you with a cloudy stock.

4. Scoop out any impurities that have gathered on the side of the pot and discard.

5. Strain through a fine-mesh strainer. Freeze any leftover stock. See Freezing Tip 30.

recipe tip: All stocks should have a mirepoix base, meaning 2 parts onion, 1 part carrot, and 1 part celery. Here, aim for 2 cups onion, 1 cup celery, and 1 cup carrot. The other 2 cups can be whatever vegetable scraps you have lying around.

beef stock

JILLIAN FORTE 🕐 **4-8 HOURS** 👥 **MAKES 3+ QUARTS** **GLUTEN-FREE** **DAIRY-FREE**

Beef stock is quite a bit different from veggie or chicken stock. The bones are roasted until the meat is very dark, which lends a caramelized flavor and a richer color to the stock. If possible, use a combination of marrow and knuckle bones, each of which adds a nuanced quality. I also add wine, and tomato paste, and go heavier on the peppercorns and woody herbs like sage and thyme. Getting a thick, dark-colored, gelatinous stock is a mark of a quality chef.

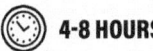 *gather*

cutting, board, chef's knife, long handled spoon, stock pot, fine mesh strainer

3-4 lbs beef bones, marrow, knuckles, shanks, feet

2 medium yellow or white onions, quartered

4 medium celery ribs, rough chopped

2 medium carrots, rough chopped

½ cup tomato paste

1 cup red wine

3 cloves garlic

4 bay leaves

1 Tbsp black peppercorns

1 tsp kosher salt

2-4 parsley stems

2-3 thyme stems

2-3 sage stems

1 gallon cold water

1. Heat the oven to 450°. Place the beef bones in a roasting pan or on an older baking sheet. Bake for 30 minutes. Chop the vegetables.

2. Add the onions, celery, and carrots to the pan. Smear the tomato paste on the beef bones. Place back into the oven for an additional 20 minutes or until the veggies are brown.

3. Place the veggies and bones into a stockpot. Pour the wine onto the still hot roasting pan or baking sheet. This will deglaze the pan and pull all the delicious caramelized flavors off the pan. Use a metal spatula to scrape up the browned bits. Pour the wine and bits into the stockpot.

4. Add the remaining ingredients to the pot. Bring to a simmer. If possible, place the stockpot half on the burner and half off. This creates a circular motion in the pot and pushes any impurities off to the side, which you can easily scoop out and discard.

5. Simmer for 4-12 hours. When done, the marrow bones should be hollow. If there is a substance inside the bones, there is more flavor to be had. Simmer the stock for another hour or until it is gone.

6. Scoop out any impurities that have gathered on the side of the pot and discard.

7. Strain the stock through a fine-mesh strainer. Freeze any leftover stock. See Freezing Tip 30. Hint: To make a simple demi-glace, add red wine and reduce the strained stock for multiple hours until the volume is reduced in half.

pro tip

Removing fat from stocks: If you are going to use the stock straight away, remove the fat before you strain it. Slowly lower a ladle into the top portion of the stock. The liquid fat on the top will stream into the ladle. Once stock enters the ladle, pull it straight up and out. Discard the oil. Repeat on a different side of the stock until most of the fat is removed. Conversely, you can completely cool the stock in the refrigerator. Once cold, the fat will coagulate on the surface and you can simply peel it away and discard it (or save it for other recipes).

chester creek tomato bisque

**JILLIAN FORTE &
MICAH NEWMAN**   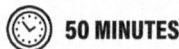 **50 MINUTES**   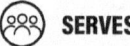 **SERVES 4**   **GLUTEN-FREE**   **VEGAN**   ***DAIRY-FREE**

Once upon a time, the kitchen crew set out to create the best tomato bisque in the Northland, one to warm in winter, refresh in summer, a soup perfect for dunking our Deluxe Grilled Cheese sandwich 64. Experimentation led to varying results, some soups were not worth giving away, some incredibly tasty, but much too complicated. In the end, we found the winning combination. It's red peppers, paprika, and orange zest that round out this bisque's fantastic flavor. As many of you know, it's a year-round pleaser.

gather

soup pot, chef knife, cutting board, liquid measuring cup, measuring spoons and cups, can opener, long-handled spoon, zester, immersion blender, or blender

1-2 tsp canola oil

¾ cup red onion, 1-inch dice (approx. ½ large)

2 tsp fresh minced garlic

¾ tsp domestic paprika

½ tsp dried, powdered rosemary

¼ tsp black pepper

¾ tsp kosher salt

1- 28 oz can plum tomatoes, peeled with basil

6 oz roasted red peppers, drained (approx. ½ jar)

1+ cups cold water

⅛ tsp orange zest (approx. ¼ orange)

¾ cup heavy cream *omit or sub for d.f.

1. Dice the red onions to approx. 1-inch. Mince the garlic.

2. Heat a heavy-bottomed soup pot on medium heat. Add the oil and wait 1 minute. Sauté the red onions for 5 minutes or until translucent. Add the garlic and sauté for one minute.

3. Add the paprika, rosemary, black pepper, and salt, in order to "bloom" them. See Pro-Tip 151. Stir for one minute or until fragrant. Add the plum tomatoes and drained red peppers. Rinse the tomato cans with 1 cup of water and pour into the soup. Turn up the heat slightly.

4. Zest about ¼ an orange into the soup. Pour in the heavy cream. Simmer for 15-20 minutes on low heat. If the soup bubbles vigorously, lower the heat.

5. Puree the soup with an immersion blender until smooth. Or, scoop 2-3 cups of soup into a kitchen blender (do not overfill) and process until smooth. Pour into a clean pot. Continue blending the soup in batches.

6. Pour the finished soup into bowls and serve with Deluxe Grilled Cheese sandwiches 64! This soup freezes well. See Freezing Tip 30.

Peters "office" - The restaurant is built on Taran's Market foundation so certain areas of the basement are not exactly level. The maintenance/storage space/Peter's office is so much like Willy Wonka's room that got shorter and shorter as you walked back. I always brought new staff there on the tour of the place. - Jillian Forte (chef)

For years, the Cafe didn't have an immersion blender large enough to puree our 5-gallon soup batches. We had to load the piping hot soup pot onto a cart and roll it through the kitchen into the coffee bar where we'd puree the soup two ladles at a time in the little blender used for making smoothies.

The blender was housed in a plastic box to keep the sound down for customers. It turns out that the plastic box had its advantages because at least once a year an impatient chef would add too much soup to the blender, causing its lid to blow. Instead of employees being sprayed with hot soup, the hot soup sprayed all over the inside of the box!

The Cafe finally purchased an immersion blender that stands about 3 feet tall. It's affectionately known as the trolling motor.

thai chicken coconut soup

JILLIAN FORTE 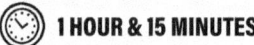 **1 HOUR & 15 MINUTES** 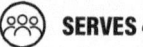 **SERVES 4**   **GLUTEN-FREE**   **DAIRY-FREE**

Crafting a terrific soup requires finding the balance between umami and acid. This recipe is good for experimentation. I love the sour zip that comes from the citrus and often play with the levels I use. This soup brings the smoothness of coconut milk and the vibrant color of the red pepper strands. It's inevitable that when I'm at the point of tasting, I typically "taste" an entire bowl! Oh, and don't skip the fish sauce. It's the magic!

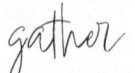 **3-4 quart soup pot, chef knife, cutting board, measuring spoons and cups, 3 small bowls, 1 larger bowl, can opener, zester, kitchen shears (optional), small strainer**

1 quart chicken stock (32 oz box or homemade)

½ medium jalapeño, minced

2 Tbsp minced shallot (approx. 1 small)

2 tsp fresh minced garlic

2 tsp fresh minced ginger

2 cups fresh shiitake caps, ¼-inch slice (approx. 2-5oz boxes)

2 cups red bell pepper, ¼-inch slice (approx. 1½ peppers)

3 Tbsp fish sauce

2- 13.5 oz cans coconut milk (not drinking type)

1 packed tsp lemon zest (approx. ¾ lemon)

1 tsp lemon juice

½ packed tsp lime zest (approx. 1 lime)

½ tsp lime juice

1+ cup baby spinach, rough chopped

2 Tbsp minced cilantro + ¼ cup whole leaves (approx. ½ bunch)

7 oz rice noodles (Thai Kitchen vermicelli thick cut)

1-2 tsp canola and sesame oil combined (optional)

8 oz chicken, raw or rotisserie chicken, 1-inch dice

kosher salt (optional)

1. Pour the chicken stock into a soup pot. Turn the heat to medium-low.

2. De-seed and mince the jalapeño pepper. Put half into the soup pot. Reserve the other half as a garnish or add in the final steps.

3. Peel and mince the shallot, garlic, and ginger and place in the soup pot.

4. Remove the stems from the shiitakes, then slice the caps to approx. ¼-inch. Add to the soup pot. Slice the red bell pepper into ¼-inch strips, then cut into 2-inch lengths. Add to the soup.

5. Add the fish sauce and coconut milk. Simmer for 20 minutes to meld the flavors.

6. Boil 4-5 quarts of water for the rice noodles.

7. Zest the lemon into a small bowl, measure, and set aside. Repeat with the lime. Reserve extra zest for the final steps. Roll the lemon and lime on the cutting board, then cut in half. Juice each into separate bowls and set aside. See Juicing Tip 27.

8. Rough chop the spinach to approx. 2-inch pieces. De-stem the cilantro. Mince 2 tablespoons and save the remaining whole leaves for garnish.

9. Cook the rice noodles in the boiling water. You can follow the instructions on the back of the noodle package or see Rice Noodle Tip 29. Once the noodles are soft but not falling apart, strain and run under cold water. Cut the noodles with kitchen shears (just a couple of snips) while they are in the strainer. Long slurpy noodles in soup are messy to eat. Do not add to the soup at this time.

10. Dice the raw or precooked chicken into 1-inch cubes. Add to the soup. Simmer for 10 minutes. Conversely, you can drop uncut raw chicken meat into the soup. Allow it to cook for 15 minutes, pull it out with tongs, dice it, and return it to the soup. This saves your cutting board and knife from getting slimy and needing to be sanitized.

11. Add the citrus zest and stir.

12. Taste the soup for a balance between savory/umami (salt and fish sauce) and brightness (acid from citrus) as well as spiciness. At this point, the broth is probably dull. Add the lime juice and taste again. It's probably closer, but not there yet. Add the lemon juice and taste again. Depending on your preference, add more fish sauce, salt, citrus juice, zest, or minced jalapeño.

13. Stir in the spinach and let it wilt. Turn off the heat and add the minced cilantro.

14. To serve, place approx. a quarter of the noodles in each bowl and ladle in the soup. Garnish with whole cilantro leaves and minced jalapeño. Offer a hot sauce for extra heat.

pro tip

If you have leftovers, keep the rice noodles separate from the soup. They will become mushy if left sitting in the soup. Instead, toss ½ teaspoon sesame oil and/or 1 teaspoon canola over the noodles and store in a sealed container. Add them when reheating.

What I learned while working in a restaurant that is supportive of local food producers has been super useful in my jobs that have followed; teaching cooking and gardening to kids, working in the food sovereignty movement and learning with native kids about indigenous/cultural food practices from leaders in the food sovereignty movement like Sean Sherman, the Sioux chef, and Brian Yazzie. - Katie Schmitz (line cook)

golden gohbi matar soup

PETER RAVINSKI **1 HOUR & 30 MINUTES** **SERVES 6**   **GLUTEN-FREE**   **VEGETARIAN**   ***VEGAN**   ***DAIRY-FREE**

In Hindi, gohbi is cauliflower and matar is peas. So while this soup sounds dramatic, it's simply named for its prominent ingredients. This soup's full-bodied flavor is classic to Indian cuisine and comes from the blending of tomatoes, cumin, and coriander. Practice blooming spices with this recipe. Experiment with upping the spice levels, especially the heat. Serve with Naan bread or try your hand at Fresh Pita Bread 80!

gather

chef knife and cutting board, 3 mixing bowls, large heavy-bottomed soup pot, liquid measuring cup, measuring spoons and cups, long-handled spoon

1 small head cauliflower, cut into florets

2 medium russet potatoes, peeled, ½-inch dice

1 small shallot, minced

1 Tbsp cumin seeds

2 tsp ground cumin

3 Tbsp + 2 tsp ground coriander

2 tsp fenugreek (optional)

2 tsp turmeric

½ tsp cayenne

¼ cup ghee or clarified butter *sub oil for d.f.

28 oz can tomato puree (3 cups)

5 cups vegetable stock

1 Tbsp +1 tsp kosher salt

1- 10 oz bag peas

2-3 Tbsp minced cilantro + ¼ cup whole leaves (approx. ½ bunch)

1. Cut the cauliflower into 1-inch florets. Some stems are OK as long as the pieces are bite-sized. Peel and dice the potato into 1-inch cubes and set aside. Peel and mince the shallot. Measure the dry spices and place them together in a bowl.

2. Heat the ghee (or oil) over medium heat in a heavy-bottomed soup pot until it slides easily across the surface of the pot. Add the dried spices and stir continuously until the oil turns golden and the spices become fragrant, approx. 2 minutes.

3. Add the cauliflower florets and potato. Fry the vegetables for approx. 5 minutes stirring frequently. Ensure every piece is covered in oil.

4. Add the shallot and cook for 1 minute.

5. Pour in the tomato puree and mix. Stop stirring and wait until the tomato puree bubbles. Simmer, occasionally stirring, for 5-10 minutes or until the fat separates from the tomato, almost circling the bubbles.

6. Add the salt and vegetable stock and stir. Simmer for 20-30 minutes.

7. Mince 2-3 tablespoons of cilantro. Set aside any extra whole leaves for a garnish.

8. Once the potatoes are soft, add the peas and minced cilantro. If using fresh peas, allow them to cook on the heat for 5-10 minutes. If using frozen, they only need 1-2 minutes. Turn off the heat and taste for salt and spice level. Adjust to taste. Serve with Naan bread or Fresh Pita Bread 80 and whole cilantro leaves.

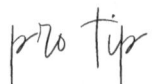

Sautéing spices in oil is a trick often employed in India. It's called "blooming" the spice. The heat releases aromatic compounds in the spice, which becomes more fragrant and powerful.

mexican caldo de res

CARLA BLUMBERG 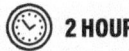 **2 HOURS** 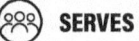 **SERVES 6** **GLUTEN-FREE** **DAIRY-FREE**

I once ordered Caldo de Res in Chiapas, Mexico. That soup's aroma, taste, and texture matched this Cafe recipe perfectly! This charming rustic soup features large hunks of vegetables, corn still on the cob, a wedge of cabbage, and meat that falls apart in your mouth. Kudos to Carla and her Texan roots for this recipe's bona fide Mexican flavor.

gather

cutting board, chef's knife, liquid measuring cup, measuring spoons, tongs, heavy-bottomed soup pot, 3-4 mixing bowls, long-handled spoon

1 medium yellow onion, 2-inch dice

8-12 oz chuck roast or fat laced cut, 1 to 2-inch cubes

1 Tbsp kosher salt

1 Tbsp black pepper

1 Tbsp canola oil

1 quart Beef Stock 146

1- 14.5 oz can plum tomatoes

2 ears corn, snapped in 3rds or 2 cups frozen

3 medium russet potatoes, 2-inch dice

3 small carrots, 2-inch dice

2 small zucchini, 2-inch dice

½ head cabbage, 1-inch wedges

2 cups water

¼ cup minced cilantro + garnish (approx. ½ bunch)

1 Tbsp +1 tsp lime Juice

12+ tortilla chips

6-8 lime wedges

1. Cut the root and stem off the onion, cut in half (root to stem), then peel. Slice each half into 3 wedges, then in half. Set aside in a bowl. Cut the beef into approx. 1-2-inch cubes. Place in a mixing bowl and sprinkle with 1 ½ teaspoon salt and 1 ½ teaspoon pepper.

2. Heat a heavy-bottomed soup pot over medium-high heat. Add the oil and wait one minute. Add half of the beef. See Pro-Tip above. Sear the beef batch by batch. Place the browned pieces in a clean bowl. Do not fully cook the beef, simply sear the outside. Once the beef is done, the pot will be very hot. Turn the heat down to medium-low. If the pot looks dry, add a teaspoon of cooking oil.

3. Add the onions, and sauté until translucent, about 4 minutes.

4. Add the beef stock, plum tomatoes, remaining salt, and pepper, and return the beef to the pot. Bring to a simmer, not a rolling boil. Cover and set a timer for 45 minutes.

5. De-husk the corn and snap each cob into 3 mini corn on the cobs (one for each serving), set aside. Peel the potatoes and carrots or scrub the skins clean. Cut each into 2-inch pieces. Place the potatoes in a bowl of water and the carrots with the corn. Slice the zucchini, cut once down the middle lengthwise, then into 2-inch pieces, set aside. Slice the cabbage into 1-2-inch wedges, keeping the stem attached to each wedge. Mince ¼ cup of cilantro. Reserve approx. ¼ cup whole leaves for garnish.

6. Once the timer goes off, add the corn, (strained) potatoes, carrots, zucchini, cabbage, and 2 cups of water. The veggies need to be covered in liquid, so add a little more water/stock if necessary or press them into the broth. Bring to a low simmer, cover, and set a timer for 30 minutes.

7. Test a piece of meat for tenderness. By now, everything should be tender. If the meat is still tight, continue simmering. Note: A lean cut of meat will rarely become extremely tender. Marbled or fatty cuts of meat melt into soft chunks.

8. Add the lime juice. Taste the soup and adjust to your preference by adding more salt or lime juice. When you find the perfect balance, turn off the heat. Add the ¼ cup minced cilantro.

9. Ladle and use tongs to divide the soup into 6 bowls, making sure each bowl has some beef, a corncob, wedge of cabbage and broth. Garnish with whole cilantro leaves, 3-4 tortilla chips nestled into the back of the bowl and lime wedges.

pro tip

Don't "crowd" the beef when searing. The meat will sweat, not sear if it is touching. This holds true for searing any type of food, particularly mushrooms and beef.

carrot ginger & quinoa soup

LYNDON RAMRATTAN **1 HOUR & 30 MINUTES** **SERVES 6**   **GLUTEN-FREE**   **VEGAN**   **DAIRY-FREE**

The appeal of this brightly colored soup is its chewy grains of quinoa, rich coconut milk, and the flavorful root powerhouses ginger and turmeric. In Ayurvedic cooking, both are considered "warming." Ginger is believed to increase circulation and aid digestion. Turmeric is lauded as an anti-inflammatory that also improves brain function. When harnessing a root's medicinal properties, fresh is best. However, raw turmeric is often difficult to find, so this recipe calls for powdered. If you can find turmeric root, mince it finely and use twice the amount listed for the powder.

gather **chef's knife and cutting board, measuring spoons, measuring cups, scale, large soup pot and small pot, long-handled spoon, immersion blender or blender**

2 lbs carrots, chopped (approx. 15 carrots)

1 ½ cups yellow onion, chopped (approx. ¾ large onion)

½ cup leek, chopped or onion (approx. ½ thin leek)

11 oz sweet potato, chopped (approx. 1 or ¾ lb)

1.5 oz fresh minced ginger (approx. 2 inches or ⅛ lb)

½ small jalapeño, minced

1 Tbsp canola oil

1 ½ tsp turmeric powder

1 tsp ground coriander

½ tsp ground cumin

2 tsp kosher salt

3 Tbsp + 2 tsp Mirin

4 ¾ cups water, divided

2 cups vegetable stock or water (not bouillon)

2 Tbsp brown sugar

1- 13.5 oz can full-fat coconut milk (Chaokoh)

½ cup quinoa

1. Chop the carrots, onions, and leeks into approx. 1-inch pieces. Size isn't that important as this is a blended soup. Peel and chop the sweet potato. Mince the ginger and set it aside. De-seed the jalapeño (or not for a spicier soup) and mince.

2. Heat a large soup pot over medium-high heat. Add the oil and wait 1 minute. Add and bloom the dried spices for 1-2 minutes. See Blooming Pro Tip 151.

3. Add the carrot, onion, and leek. Sauté for 10 minutes or until the onions are translucent. Deglaze the pot with the Mirin. Add 4 cups of water and 2 cups of vegetable stock.

4. Add the jalapeño, sweet potato, ginger, brown sugar, and coconut milk. Cover and simmer for 30 minutes.

5. Put ¾ cup of water and the quinoa into a small pot. Bring to a simmer. Cover, lower the heat, and cook for approx. 15 minutes. Stir mid-way through. The quinoa is done when the white spots are gone from the kernels. If the water is gone but there are still white spots, add 1+ tablespoon of water, stir, cover and turn off the heat. The residual heat will gently finish cooking the quinoa.

6. Once all the vegetables in the soup are soft, puree the soup. Use an immersion blender until smooth. Or, scoop 2-3 cups of soup into a kitchen blender (do not overfill) and process until smooth, pour into a clean pot. Continue blending the soup in batches until done.

7. Stir the cooked quinoa into the soup. Taste and adjust to your preference. This soup is supposed to be a touch sweet so do not over-salt.

pro tip

Rinse the quinoa before cooking it. Try using a reusable coffee filter so the small grains don't slip through your normal strainer. Don't have a scale at home? Weigh the sweet potato and ginger at the grocery store.

curried winter squash soup

RITA B BERGSTADT **1 HOUR & 15 MINUTES** **SERVES 4**   **VEGETARIAN**   **GLUTEN-FREE**   ***VEGAN**   ***DAIRY-FREE**

Northern gardeners will appreciate this soup. Choose a golden, green, or orange winter squash and a couple of fall apples. If you can harvest any of these ingredients from your yard, all the sweeter! Swirled with cream and garnished with crispy sage, this sweet curried puree will look as elegant as it tastes.

gather

chef knife, cutting board, baking sheet or medium-sized pot, an apple peeler-corer-slicer contraption, 3-4 quart soup pot, long-handled spoon, measuring cups and spoons, can opener, mixing bowl, whisk, small sauce pot, tongs, paper towels, immersion blender or blender

4 cups cooked winter squash

2 medium apples, peeled, cored, sliced, or ¾ cup applesauce

1 Tbsp unsalted butter *sub oil for d.f.

2 cups water

1- 13.5 oz can coconut milk

1+ Tbsp mild red curry paste (Pataks)

salt to taste

½ cup sour cream *sub vegan sour cream for d.f.

2 Tbsp milk or cream *sub coconut milk for d.f.

4-8 fresh sage leaves (optional)

½ - 1 cup canola oil

1. Cook the squash. You can do this ahead of time. There are many methods for cooking squash. Here are two. (1) Cut the squash in half, scoop out the seeds, and place flesh side down on a baking sheet. Add about ½ cup of water to the sheet pan and bake for approx. 40 minutes or until soft at 400°. Add more time if needed. This method enhances the sweetness of the squash and makes it easy to scoop the flesh from the skin. (2) Cut the squash in half, scoop out the seeds, peel, cut the flesh into chunks, and simmer in a pot of water until soft. This method is quicker and leaves you with flavorful water that you can use in the soup. However, it requires peeling the squash when it is raw, which can be difficult.

2. Measure out 4 cups of cooked flesh and set aside.

3. Peel, core, and slice the apples. If you have a handy gadget that does all three, perfect!

4. Melt 1 tablespoon of butter in a soup pot over medium heat. Add the apple pieces, and sauté until soft. Add the squash, water, coconut milk, and 1 tablespoon of curry paste (you can add more curry at the end). Simmer for 20 minutes.

5. Combine the sour cream and a splash of milk or cream in a mixing bowl with a fork or whisk. Set aside.

6. Heat ½ - 1 cup canola oil in a small sauté pan or sauce pot to just below the smoking point. Place 2-3 whole fresh sage leaves into it. They should sizzle and fry. Pull them out with tongs and place them on paper towels to drip dry. Repeat until all the sage is fried. Let the oil cool, then place it into a jar and label it as sage oil. Note: The flavored oil will be subtle, but you don't want to forget about this treasure. Use it in a salad dressing!

7. Puree the soup with an immersion, or kitchen, blender until smooth, almost glossy. Taste the soup for spiciness and sweetness. Sometimes a tiny pinch of salt, a splash of maple syrup, or more curry is just what it needs.

8. Ladle the soup into 4 bowls. Drizzle the sour cream mixture on the top (try a circle then drag a toothpick through it to create a heart shape). Place 1-2 fried sage leaves on top. Freeze any remaining soup and gently reheat it at a later date. See Freezing Tip 30.

recipe tips:

Kobocha, Blue Hubbard, Buttercup, or other bumpy squash have firm flesh and thick skin. The tough, thick skin makes it difficult to remove. Therefore, it is my opinion that it's best to bake and then scoop out the flesh. If you want to boil these varieties, use a knife to peel, not a vegetable peeler.

Pumpkins, Butternut, and Kuri squash have a softer texture and are easy to peel using a vegetable peeler. For this recipe, they work well boiled. If you prefer the bake and scoop method, bake at 425° or higher, which will blister the skin and help it pull away from the flesh.

roasted corn poblano chowder

JILLIAN FORTE 1 HOUR & 30 MINUTES SERVES 6-8 VEGETARIAN *GLUTEN-FREE *DAIRY-FREE

This creamy chowder is magnificent, bursting with the flavors and colors of the southwest, but slightly adjusted for the Minnesota palate. Blistered and charred red and poblano peppers, sweet, caramelized corn, and a kiss of lime juice, make this a scoop-able soup. There are a few tricks here, so pay attention to the instructions and you'll nail it every time.

gather **tongs, mixing bowl, plastic wrap, chef's knife, cutting board, liquid measuring cup, measuring cups measuring spoons, baking sheet, soup pot, long-handled spoon, sauté pan, whisk, rubber spatula**

1 poblano pepper, charred, ½-inch dice

2 red peppers, charred, sub for a can of roasted red peppers ½-inch dice

½ cup diced celery, ½-inch

2 cups diced white onion, ½-inch (approx. 1 lg)

4 cups diced baby potatoes, ½-inch (approx. 6-8 potatoes)

1½ tsp fresh minced garlic

½ medium jalapeño, minced

1 tsp canola oil

1½ cups corn kernels (approx. 2 corn cobs)

2 Tbsp +1 tsp salted butter, divided *sub oil for d.f.

4 cups vegetable stock

2 tsp kosher salt

¼ cup all-purpose flour *omit for g.f.

1 cup cold milk *sub milk alternative for d.f.

1 avocado, ½-inch dice

2 Tbsp minced cilantro

1 tsp lime juice

24-30 tortilla chips, garnish (optional)

1 cup shredded cheddar or Monterey jack cheese, garnish (optional)

1. Ignite the flames of a gas stove top, outside grill, or broil setting in an oven. Using tongs, place the poblano and red peppers directly onto the flame of the stove or grill. When one side gets black, rotate the pepper. Continue until it is charred all around. (Gray coloring signals too long on the flame. Turn quickly.) If broiling, place the peppers on a sheet pan as close to the heat as possible. Turn peppers when blistered. Blister every side. Place finished peppers in a bowl and cover tightly with plastic wrap. The steam will help the skins rub off.

2. Dice the celery and onion into ½-inch pieces and set aside together in a mixing bowl. Dice the potatoes into ½-inch cubes. Peel then mince the garlic. Slice the jalapeño in half, de-seed (or not, for a spicier soup), and mince half of it.

3. Caramelize the corn. If you are using frozen corn, turn the oven on to broil. Oil a sheet pan. Place the corn in a tight but not overlapping pile in the middle of the pan. Bake for 4-5 minutes, or until the corn is brown. You may need to give it a stir once and add more time. If using corn on the cob, lucky you! Grill it outside or use the broil setting in the oven. Rotate as the sides turn golden brown. Cool, then cut the corn from the cob by standing the cob on its flat stem side and sliding your knife from the top down. Don't use your best knife, as accidentally cutting into the cob will dull it quickly.

4. Melt 1 teaspoon of butter (or oil) in a heavy-bottomed soup pot over medium heat. Add the celery and onions and cook for 5 minutes or until soft. Add the garlic and cook for 1-2 minutes.

5. Add the jalapeño, stock, potatoes, corn, and salt. Bring to a simmer, cover, and set a timer for 30 minutes.

6. Unwrap the bowl with the peppers and work one pepper at a time. Remove the blistered skin, stem, seeds, and pith inside. Dice into ½-inch squares, then add to the soup. See Recipe Tip above.

7. Melt 2 tablespoons of butter in a sauté pan over medium-high heat. Whisk in the flour. Switch to a silicone rubber spatula and stir until the flour turns golden brown. (This is the roux that will thicken the soup.) Transfer the roux to a plate and chill in the fridge. Note: Be careful not to get the roux on your skin. It will leave nasty burns. It's almost as bad as caramelized sugar.

8. When the potatoes in the soup are soft all the way through, whisk just the top of the soup as you pour in the cold milk. Add the cold roux. Continue whisking until all the lumps are dissolved. Why cold roux? See Pro Tip below.

9. Bring the soup to a boil to activate the roux. Occasionally scrape the bottom and edges of the pot with a spatula as flour can sink and stick.

10. Roughly de-stem, then mince the cilantro. Cut the avocado in half, remove the pit, scoop out the flesh, and dice to ½-inch. See Avocado Cutting Tip 29.

11. Stir in the diced avocado, cilantro, and lime juice. Taste and adjust by adding more salt, lime juice, or jalapeño as desired. Serve with 4-5 tortilla chips tucked in each bowl and 2 tablespoons of shredded cheese sprinkled on top.

recipe tip: Peel and remove the seeds from charred peppers in a sink. Run a thin stream of water in your sink to occasionally rinse your hands of the sticky seeds and skins. Try not to rinse the peppers themselves, thus preserving their flavor.

pro tip

Roux, a classic thickener, will occasionally separate into fat and flour and not "work". The trick to ensure a roux does not break is to have either the liquid (the soup), or the roux be cold. In this case, we chill the roux before adding it to the hot soup. Other recipes, such as the Basic Kids Mac N Cheese & Adult Mac 89 call for cold liquids to be whisked into a hot roux.

veggie loaded beef stew

JILLIAN FORTE 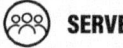 1 HOUR & 30 MINUTES SERVES 3-4 *GLUTEN-FREE DAIRY-FREE

A good beef stew purrs comfort and contentment. As a child, I was a picky eater and leaned toward vegetarianism, but I often craved canned beef stew. I'd open the can and mine it for the vegetables, slipping the chunks of meat to our dog. True to my roots, this stew features more veggies than meat. Use high-quality beef stock for a rich, deep flavor, or better yet, make your own 146! Serve with your favorite bread, slathered in real butter to soak up all the good stuff.

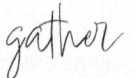 chef's knife, cutting board, mixing bowls, large high-sided cast iron, or a heavy-bottomed pot or Dutch oven, liquid measuring cup, dry measuring cups, measuring spoons, silicone spatula, fork, or small whisk

8 oz crimini mushrooms, quartered

½ yellow onion, julienned

1 clove garlic, sliced

1 large carrot, 1-inch dice

2 medium red potatoes, 1-inch dice

1 parsnip or ¼ rutabaga, peeled, 1-inch dice

8-12 oz chuck roast, 1-inch dice

¼ tsp black pepper

1 ½ tsp kosher salt

3-4+ Tbsp bacon fat or butter

1 Tbsp tomato paste

¼ cup all-purpose flour *omit for g.f.

¼ cup red wine

4 cups Beef Stock 146

1 tsp g.f. tamari

¼ tsp Worcestershire

2 bay leaves

4-5 twigs fresh thyme

1 sprig fresh sage

1 sprig fresh parsley

2 cups peas

1. Quarter or halve the crimini mushrooms, and set aside in a medium-sized bowl. Julienne the yellow onion, then halve the strips. Add to the bowl. Peel then slice the garlic clove, and set aside in a small bowl. Peel (or not), and dice the carrot, potatoes, and parsnips into 1-inch cubes. Set these aside together in a third bowl. Note: If you are not cooking immediately, cover the potatoes in water to prevent discoloration.

2. Trim off any large pieces of silver skin from the beef, then dice it into 1-inch cubes. Place in a mixing bowl and sprinkle with the salt and pepper.

3. Melt 1 tablespoon of bacon fat in the soup pot over medium-high heat. Add half of the beef and sear it on all sides, not fully cooked. Don't let the pieces touch as they will sweat instead of sear. As pieces finish, remove, and place in a clean bowl. The pot will get hotter and hotter. You can gradually reduce the heat so nothing scorches. Continue until all the pieces are seared and set aside.

4. Add another tablespoon of bacon fat or butter to the pot. If it smokes, remove the pan from the heat and let it cool down for 2-3 minutes before continuing. Add the mushrooms and onions, then sauté for approx. 5 minutes. Once the onions are soft, add the garlic and cook for one minute.

5. Add the tomato paste and mix until it coats the vegetables.

6. Push all the vegetables off to one side of the pan or transfer them to a clean bowl. Drop a generous tablespoon of bacon fat or butter in the open spot. Once melted, sprinkle the flour over the butter. Continuously stir the mixture with a silicone rubber spatula until it turns light brown. Try to keep this mini roux confined to the open space.

7. Pour the wine on top of the roux while mixing with a fork or whisk so it doesn't clump. Pour the beef stock in and mix. Completely integrate the roux into the stock with a whisk.

8. Add the Worcestershire and tamari, and mix well.

9. Nestle the beef, carrots, potatoes, and parsnips into the stock. If you removed the mushrooms and onions, return them to the pan now.

10. Place the bay leaves and fresh herbs on top of the stew. Ensure the vegetables, beef, and herbs are submerged in the liquid. Use a spatula to press everything down, or add a bit more stock if needed.

11. Bring the stew up to a bubbling simmer. This will kick start the roux. Lower the temperature, cover, and set a timer for 30 minutes. You may need more time for the beef to soften up, but 30 is a good place to start.

12. Uncover the stew and test the broth for flavor. Now is the time to add a bit more tamari or salt if needed. Fish out the bay leaves and fresh herb sprigs and discard. If little bits are in the stew that is OK, but no one enjoys finding a 7-inch long parsley stem hanging out of their mouth!

13. Add the peas and stir. If the peas are fresh, they will need about 5-10 minutes to cook. If they are frozen, then they simply need to be heated. Served with warm bread and real butter.

pro tip

Parsnips, and turnips, are often preserved in a coat of wax. Remove the protective layer by flaking it off by hand, or by soaking them in hot water for 3-5 minutes. Or use a vegetable brush to scrape off the wax, then rinse it under hot water. Peel the parsnip to ensure all the wax is gone. On the other hand, carrots and/or potatoes do not need to be peeled. For an earthy flavor and higher mineral content, give them a good scrub under running water and skip the peeling.

pork pho noodle bowl

CARLA BLUMBERG **7 ½ - 13 HOURS** 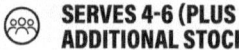 **SERVES 4-6 (PLUS ADDITIONAL STOCK)** **DAIRY-FREE** **GLUTEN-FREE**

The joy and pleasure of Pho is derived from its broth. This slurp-able broth, though long-simmering, is a breeze. Roast the bones and veggies in the morning, then simmer them throughout the day in a large stockpot. Dinner time requires straining and spicing the broth, cooking the meat, and light prep. This stock recipe will make enough for 2-3 meals, as it is difficult to source half a pig trotter. Freeze the extra for use another time or other soup.

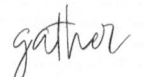

two baking pans, chef's knife, cutting board, cast iron or sauté pan, large stockpot or large roasting pan, aluminum foil, boning knife, mixing bowl, plastic wrap, measuring spoons, measuring cups, zester, Sous Vide machine (optional), medium-sized pot, strainer, box grater

STOCK

1 pig trotter, ham hock, or shank

1 lb chicken bones
(ask the butcher)

3 whole yellow onions, quartered

5 oz fresh shiitake mushrooms

½ head fennel, chopped

2-3 medium carrots, chopped

4-5 celery stalks, chopped

5 quarts cold water

1 ½ cups fresh ginger, chopped

3 cloves fresh garlic, smashed

1 stalk lemongrass, chopped

¼ cup star anise

1 cinnamon stick

1-2 pods cardamom (optional

🔔 Optional to make 1-3 days ahead.

1. Heat the oven to 375°. Bake the pig trotters and chicken bones on a lightly greased baking sheet for 30 minutes.

2. Peel and quarter the onions. Rough chop the fennel, carrots, and celery stalks. Place the veggies and mushrooms on a second lightly greased sheet pan. When the timer goes off, place the veggies in the oven with the bones and set the timer for an additional 30 minutes.

3. Rough chop the ginger into 1-inch pieces. Lay your knife flat side down on the ginger and press firmly to smash them. Smash the unpeeled garlic cloves, then peel. Rough chop the lemon grass. Set the aromatics asid e together in a bowl.

4. Toast the star anise, cinnamon stick, and cardamom in a dry cast iron or sauté pan for 4 minutes or until fragrant. Slide these into the bowl with the ginger, lemongrass, and garlic.

SIMMERING THE STOCK-TWO OPTIONS

A. The stove top option. Place the bones, vegetables, and aromatics into a large stockpot, add 5 quarts of water (1 ¼ gallon), and put on the stovetop on low heat. Simmer for 6-10 hours. The stock needs to be slightly bubbling. If possible, set the stock pot on the edge of the burner. This creates a circular effect as the water gently rolls around the pot, pushing impurities off to one side, which you can easily remove with a spoon. This offset simmer also ensures that the stock does not boil rapidly. Note: A vigorously boiling stock can become cloudy as the fats emulsify into the broth. If you can't seem to adjust the heat to a slight bubble, cover ¾ of the pot with aluminum foil so the liquid doesn't evaporate.

B. The oven option. Heat the oven to 225°. Place the bones, vegetables, aromatics, and water in a roasting pan. Tightly seal with aluminum foil, then put it in the oven for 8-12 hours. This is a simpler and more flexible method. However, most of us don't have a roasting pan large enough for these ingredients. It is possible that your large stock pot will fit in the oven with all the shelves removed, which is an acceptable option as long as you remember that the handles are very hot.

PORK MARINADE

1 pork tenderloin

¼ cup canola oil

2 Tbsp lemon juice

2 Tbsp fresh minced garlic

2 Tbsp fresh minced ginger

1 Tbsp kosher salt

2 tsp mustard powder

½ tsp Cubeb pepper or ground allspice

🔔 Optional to make 1-2 days ahead.

1. Remove the silver skin from the pork tenderloin. See Pro Tip above.

2. Whisk the oil, lemon juice, garlic, ginger, salt, mustard powder, and Cubeb pepper or allspice in a mixing bowl.

3. Place the trimmed tenderloins in the marinade and completely coat the loin. Cover the bowl with plastic wrap, pushing it down so no air touches the pork. If you have a Sous Vide machine, place the pork and marinade into one of the cooking bags, remove oxygen, and seal. The sous vide method takes over 2 ½ hours to cook, so plan ahead. To Sous Vide or not to Sous Vide? See some pros and cons 30.

4. Place in the fridge for a minimum of 6 hours and a maximum of 48 hours.

> ## pro Tip
>
> Remove the silver skin that envelops a pork tenderloin with a thin flexible boning knife. Push the blade into the pork just beneath the silver skin, with the blade tilted slightly towards the "skin". Slide the blade along the meat, freeing the tough part from the tender flesh. Repeat until it is all removed and discard the trimmings.

FINALE

2 Tbsp g.f. fish sauce

1 tsp lime zest

¼ cup g.f. tamari

1- 14 oz pack rice noodles, thick cut

2 cups mung bean sprouts

1 cup shredded carrot (approx. 2 carrots)

¼ cup green onions, thinly sliced (approx. 1-2)

1 cup snow peas

20 leaves Thai basil

20 leaves fresh mint

¼ cup crushed peanuts

1 lime, wedged

1. Heat the oven to 400° or set the Sous Vide water circulator to 136°.

2. Strain the stock through a fine-mesh strainer into a clean pot. Discard the bones, veggies, and aromatics.

3. Add the fish sauce, lime zest, and tamari. Adjust to your preference by adding more tamari, fish sauce, or lime juice. You are looking for a balance here, use your critical thinking and play with your food! The stock is ready but should stay on the stovetop to hold its heat.

4. Cook the pork tenderloin in the oven for 20 minutes or in a Sous Vide water bath for 2 hours and 35 minutes. The internal temperature should be 145 for the oven and 136 for Sous Vide. A little pink is good! Slice the pork into ¼ - ½-inch circles and set aside.

5. While the pork is cooking, bring a pot of water to a boil. Cook the noodles according to the package or see Rice Noodle Tip 29. Once the noodles are soft but not falling apart, strain and portion into 4 bowls. Extra noodles? See Tip 150.

6. Shred the carrots on a box grater. Thinly slice the green onions, de-stem the snow peas, pick the fresh basil and mint leaves, and cut the limes into wedges. Rough chop the peanuts.

7. To assemble, put the rice noodles into each of the four bowls, pour the broth over the noodles, place a quarter of the pork into each bowl and a portion of each of the garnishes on top. Serve with lime wedges, a hot sauce of your choosing, and a bowl of crushed peanuts.

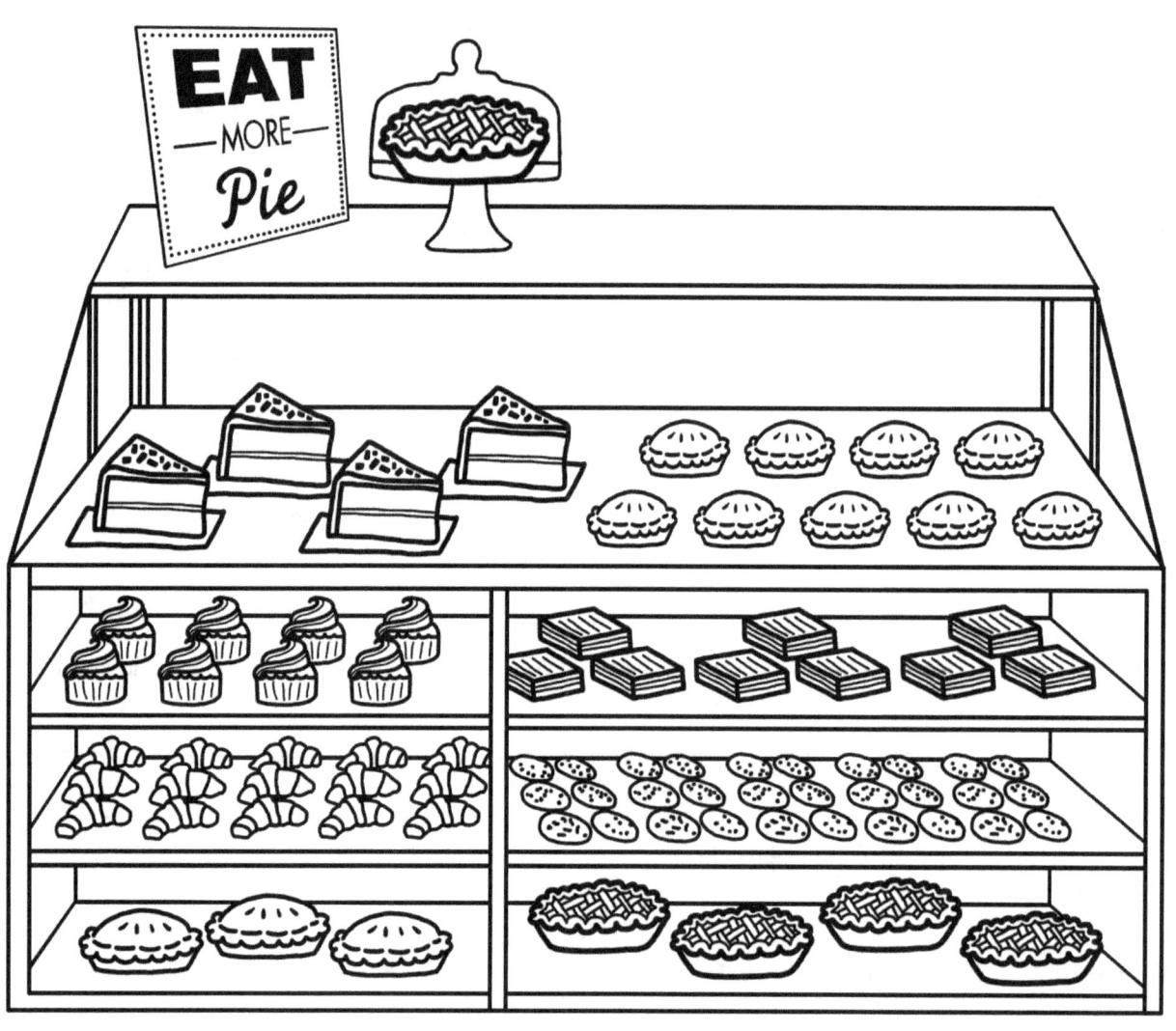

ILLUSTRATED BY: AMANDA CLARK (*SERVER, GRAPHIC DESIGNER*)

baked desserts

Anyone who has walked into At Sara's Table Chester Creek Cafe knows the bakery is eye-catching. Displayed in the case are glossy brownies, freshly baked scones with their light reflecting sanding sugar, the beckoning deep pinks of a strawberry-rhubarb pie. Inevitably, there's an item that pulls at me, tugging at my desire for dessert before dinner.

Diane Bailey, our baker for 18 years, had a grandmother's touch for offering comfort through food. It was her skill and charm that created the bakery our restaurant is famous for. It was her Gluten-Free offerings that started our journey toward an allergy aware kitchen. This section's selections include a G.F. & Vegan Brownie and a substitution for the Morning Glory based on our oat flour mix. (A second G.F. flour mix is in this book's Breakfast section.) Try preparing, then baking, fresh scones in the morning like the Cafe. It's an excellent way to start the day. The Cafe's Apricot Rugelach is my favorite, small portioned and perfectly sweet. Baking requires patience and practice, but the only thing better than eating a sugary mistake is devouring sweet perfection!

morning glory muffins

DIANE BAILEY 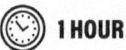 1 HOUR & 21 MINUTES YIELDS 18 MUFFINS   VEGETARIAN   *GLUTEN-FREE

Muffins. The guilt-free cousins of cupcakes. Or so I like to believe! These Morning Glory Muffins are made with fruit, nuts, and carrots, therefore "healthy" sweet. At the Cafe we baked them with coarse sugar granules on top. Like many people, I eat that part first!

gather

three mixing bowls, chef knife, cutting board, vegetable peeler, box grater, measuring cups, measuring spoons, wooden spoon or rubber spatula, zester, whisk, muffin pans and corresponding sized muffin cups usually 2 ½ inch

½ cup craisins, re-hydrated

½ cup walnuts, chopped

½ cup shredded coconut

1 ⅓ cup apples, ¼-inch dice (approx. 1 large)

2 cups carrots, shredded (approx. 2)

2 cups all-purpose flour *sub Oat Flour Dry Mix 172

1 ½ cups white sugar

¼ tsp ground cinnamon

¼ tsp ground nutmeg

¼ scant tsp ground allspice

½ tsp iodized salt

1 ⅛ tsp baking soda

3 eggs

⅔ cup + 1 Tbsp Canola oil

2 tsp vanilla extract

1 tsp orange zest

¼-½ cup sanding sugar

1. Heat the convection or conventional oven to 325°.

2. Rehydrate the craisins in scalding tap water. Chop the walnuts to ¼-inch or smaller. Peel, then dice the apple into ¼-inch pieces. Peel, then shred the carrot on a box grater. Set aside together in a mixing bowl.

3. Add the shredded coconut to the bowl.

4. In a separate bowl, mix the flour, sugar, cinnamon, nutmeg, all-spice, salt, and baking soda. Pour the dry mix over the fruits and veggies. Mix thoroughly.

5. Crack and whisk the eggs into a third mixing bowl. Add the oil, vanilla, and orange zest. Whisk until uniform, then pour over the mixed ingredients. Combine with a wooden spoon.

6. Evenly divide the batter into lined muffin tins. Standard size tins (2 ½ inches), will make 18 muffins. Sprinkle each muffin with sanding sugar.

7. Bake for 15 minutes. Then lower the temp to 315° and bake for an additional 12 minutes. Use a toothpick to ensure the cupcakes are done before allowing them to cool. See Toothpick Pro Tip 164.

pro tip

Individually wrap extra, cooled muffins tightly in plastic wrap, then freeze them. They make a great breakfast on the run. Simply take one out of the freezer the night before and it will be ready to eat by morning!

oatmeal chocolate chip cookies

DIANE BAILEY 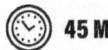 **45 MINUTES** **YIELDS 15 COOKIES** **VEGETARIAN**

These cookies are thick and hearty, perfect for a midday snack, or dessert after a light meal. Plus, there's oatmeal in them, so they're kind of healthy, right?!

gather

two mixing bowls, electric beater, measuring spoons and cups, rubber spatula, baking sheet, 3oz scoop

½ cup unsalted butter, softened

¼ cup brown sugar, packed

¼ cup white sugar

1 tsp milk

1 egg

½ tsp vanilla extract

1 cup rolled oats

½ cup all-purpose flour

¼ cup whole wheat pastry flour

½ tsp baking soda

½ tsp iodized salt

¾ cup chocolate chips

pan spray or butter to grease the pan

1. Heat the convection oven to 325°. A conventional oven to 400°.

2. Cream the butter and sugars together in a mixing bowl with an electric beater.

3. Add the milk, egg, and vanilla. Blend until combined.

4. Mix the oats, flours, baking soda, and salt in a separate mixing bowl. Pour into the wet ingredients and mix.

5. Add the chocolate chips and mix. Place in the refrigerator for 20-30 minutes to chill the dough.

6. Using the pan spray or butter, grease the baking sheet or use parchment paper. Scoop 3 oz (approx. 3 tablespoons) of the dough onto the baking sheet. Leave room for the cookies to expand while baking. Slightly press the cookie dough down to help with even baking.

7. Bake for 15 minutes, then rotate the pan 180 degrees and bake for an additional 10 minutes. Test the cookies using the toothpick method.

pro tip

Toothpick method - Poke a toothpick into the thickest part of baked goods and pull it out. If there is dough stuck to the toothpick, it is not done cooking. If it slides out clean, then they are ready to go.

scones
RASPBERRY WHITE CHOCOLATE OR BLUEBERRY OR CRANBERRY ORANGE

**DIANE BAILEY &
RITA B BERGSTEDT**

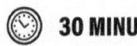 30 MINUTES

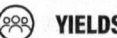 YIELDS 8 SCONES

VEGETARIAN

Unlike the Cafe customers, the staff enters through the building's back door and head to the basement locker area, which shares the same floor as the bakery. Being greeted on sleepy early mornings by the sweet scent of caramelized sugar and baked blueberries is like being enveloped in a warm hug. Scones right out of the oven are a simple pleasure. In order to have fresh ones daily, Diane designed a large-batch recipe that allowed for freezing the dough triangles and baking off just the right amount. This recipe makes 8. If your desire is for fewer, follow Diane's lead and freeze some dough for another day.

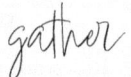 **food processor, two mixing bowls, spatula, measuring spoons and cups, bench/pastry knife, baking sheet, parchment paper or silicone mat**

DOUGH

2 cups all-purpose flour (10.6 oz)

5 Tbsp white sugar

1 ½ tsp baking powder

½ tsp iodized salt

5 Tbsp +1 ½ tsp cold unsalted butter

1 egg

¾ cup heavy cream

1. Heat the oven to 425°.

2. Combine the flour, sugar, baking powder, and salt in a food processor.

3. Cut the butter into 1-inch chunks and drop them into the flour mixture. Pulse until the butter is pea-sized, approx. ¼ -inch. Transfer to a mixing bowl.

4. In a second mixing bowl, whisk together the cream and the egg. Set aside.

5. Follow the directions below for your filling choice.

RASPBERRY WHITE CHOCOLATE

¾ cups raspberries,
fresh or frozen

¼ cup white chocolate chips

½ shot Torani raspberry syrup or raspberry jam

1. Stir the fresh or defrosted raspberries and white chocolate chips into the dough. Combine the Torani raspberry syrup with ¼ cup of the egg and cream mixture from step 4 above. Add this mixture to the dough in step 1 below.

BLUEBERRY

⅜ tsp ground cardamom

¾ tsp lemon zest
(approx. ½ lemon)

¾ cup blueberries,
fresh or frozen

1. Stir the cardamom into the flour in step 2. Stir the lemon zest and blueberries into the dough. Hint: If using frozen blueberries, allow them to defrost in a strainer to remove excess liquid.

CRANBERRY-ORANGE

1 cup cranberries,
rehydrated

2 Tbsp + 1 tsp orange zest (approx. 2 oranges)

1. Rehydrate the cranberries in scalding tap water before you start step one above. Strain the cranberries and pat dry. Stir the cranberries and orange zest into the dough.

FINISHING

1. Add approx. ¼ cup of the egg-cream mixture to the dough and fillings. Mix with a spatula until the dough just comes together. If it needs more liquid, add approx. 1 tablespoon at a time. Do not over-mix. Set aside the remaining wet mixture for brushing the tops of the scones.

2. Transfer the dough onto a clean and floured work surface. Press together to form a rough ball. Flatten into a disk with your hands, fold in half and flatten again. Repeat 4-5 times. Note: We are trying to add layers of air, therefore gently pat each layer.

3. Flatten the dough into a 7-inch circle, ¾-inch thick. Using the bench knife, cut the circle into 8 even wedges.

   🔔 If you want to freeze the dough to be cooked off later, stop here. Place the dough triangles (untouching) on a lined baking sheet and place them in the freezer. When frozen, transfer them to a zip-top baggie and keep them stored in the freezer. On the day you would like to bake them, defrost for approx. 20 minutes before baking. They may take slightly longer than the fresh ones to bake.

4. Place each wedge on a parchment-lined baking sheet with room for each to expand. Brush the tops with the cream-egg mixture and sprinkle with coarse sugar.

5. Bake at 425° for 15 minutes or until golden brown. Enjoy!

apricot or almond rugelach

DIANE BAILEY **2 HOURS & 45 MINUTES** **YIELDS 12 RUGELACH** **VEGETARIAN**

All the baked goods at the Cafe are dated for freshness and then pulled from the bakery case if not sold. As you can imagine, these are happy moments for the staff. I kept my eye out for the rare unsold rugelach. Discovering one (before my cohorts) was a moment to give thanks! I would stow my treasure until my break and then savor every crunchy, sweet bite. This recipe is a bit persnickety. It's important to use sliced almonds and to resist the temptation to overfill the dough. Choose between Apricot or Almond filling. My favorite is the apricot, which also is easier.

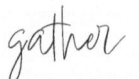 food processor, wax paper, chef knife and cutting board, rolling pin, pizza wheel, sheet pan, parchment paper or silicone mat

DOUGH

1 cup all-purpose flour (5.3 oz)

½ tsp iodized salt

10 ½ Tbsp cold, unsalted butter

⅓ cup sour cream

¾ cup sliced almonds, finely chopped

1 cup white sugar

1. Combine the flour and salt in the bowl of a food processor. Pulse 2 times to blend.

2. Cut the cold butter into the flour mixture. Pulse 5-6 times until the butter is pea-sized, approx. ¼ inch. Add the sour cream and pulse an additional 4-5 times.

3. Remove the dough onto a lightly floured work surface and shape it into a 1-inch thick patty. Wrap in wax paper and place in the fridge for at least 2 hours. Hint: If you do not wait two hours, the dough will fall apart while baking.

🔔 If making the Almond Filling, start now. It also needs to be chilled.

APRICOT FILLING

¼ cup apricot jam

ALMOND FILLING

4 Tbsp unsalted butter

2 cups sliced almonds, finely chopped

1 egg

½ cup white sugar

¼ tsp iodized salt

1 tsp lemon zest, puree, or fresh

¼ tsp almond extract

1. Melt the butter and pour it into a mixing bowl.

2. Mince 2 cups of sliced almonds to ⅛-inch or smaller.

3. Whisk the egg with the butter until uniform. Add the almonds and remaining ingredients to the mixing bowl. Stir well to combine and place in the refrigerator until ready to use.

FINISHING

1. Heat a convection oven to 325°. A conventional oven to 350°.

2. Mince ¾ cup sliced almonds to ⅛-inch or smaller.

3. Mix the almonds with the sugar in a bowl. Sprinkle your work surface with 2-3 tablespoons of this mixture. Place the dough on top and roll out a circle, approx. 6-inches in diameter. If the dough is sticking to the surface, gently lift it and sprinkle more sugar-almond mixture beneath.

4. Lift the dough and sprinkle another 2-3 tablespoons of the sugar-almond mix on the table. Flip the dough, then roll it out into a 12-inch wide circle.

5. Cut the circle into even fourths using a pizza wheel. Cut each quarter into 3 even wedges, yielding 12 triangles.

6. Place approx. 1 teaspoon of either apricot jam or Almond Filling on the wide end of each wedge, but not touching the edges. Starting at the wide end, roll each wedge into a croissant. Make sure the tip is under the roll at the end. Bend into a crescent moon shape and coat with the sugar-almond mixture.

7. Chill prepared rugelach on a parchment-lined baking sheet for 20 minutes.

8. Place the rugelach into the oven on the middle shelf. Bake until puffed up and a golden brown, approx. 20 minutes rotate the pan at the 10-minute mark.

9. Remove the rugelach to a wire cooling rack so they do not become fused to the parchment paper as they cool. They can be served once cool to the touch and up to 5 days later if stored in the fridge.

One day when Katie Schmitz (line cook) was mixing the flour, she turned on the machine, which was set to 3 instead of 1, and in a single poof, the white flour covered her from head to black chef coat to toe!

brownies with fudge frosting

DIANE BAILEY **1 HOUR & 10 MINUTES** **YIELDS 12 BROWNIES**

This recipe adds fudge to an already moist brownie, making it a chocolate lover's dream come true! Use high-quality cocoa powder and chocolate chips to recreate this well-loved dessert at home. I like to add walnuts for textural variety, though I know some of you prefer your chocolate unadulterated. One mysterious fact, these brownies are even better on the second day!

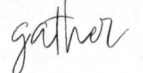 whisk or electric beaters, 2 mixing bowls, measuring spoons and cups, 9 x 13-inch baking pan, wooden spoon, rubber spatula, medium-sized saucepan (preferably heavy-bottomed)

BROWNIES

2 ½ sticks unsalted butter (1 ¼ cup)

¾ cup white sugar

1 cup brown sugar, packed

½ tsp iodized salt

½ cup cocoa powder (Valrhona)

1 ½ tsp vanilla extract

4 eggs

1 cup all-purpose flour

pan spray, butter

1 cup walnuts, chopped (optional)

1. Heat the oven to 325°. Melt the butter.

2. Using an electric beater, cream both sugars, salt, cocoa powder, vanilla, and butter.

3. In a separate bowl, whisk the eggs until well beaten. Pour into the sugar mix and stir with a rubber spatula. If you are adding walnuts, mix them into the batter now. Set aside a few tablespoons of the nuts to sprinkle on the top of the frosted brownie.

4. Fold the flour into the mixture. Do not over-mix.

5. Spray a 9 x 13-inch baking pan with butter spray or rub a stick of cool butter over the bottom and side of the pan. Hint: You can sprinkle a little flour into the pan and shake it to cover the butter. Dump out any loose flour. This will help your brownies to lift cleanly from the pan.

6. Pour the batter into the pan. Use a spatula to spread out the batter, slightly pushing more batter to the corners and edges.

7. Bake for 40 minutes. Use the Toothpick Pro Tip 164 to ensure the brownies are done cooking. Cool for about 20 minutes, then start the fudge frosting!

FUDGE FROSTING

5 Tbsp milk

¾ cup white sugar

1 pinch iodized salt

6 Tbsp unsalted butter

1 cup chocolate chips, semi-sweet

1 tsp vanilla extract

½ cup walnuts, chopped (optional)

1. Pour the milk, sugar, salt, and butter into the saucepan. Turn the heat to medium-high. Measure out the chocolate chips and vanilla and have them waiting near the saucepan.

2. Boil the mixture for 1 minute. Add the chocolate chips and vanilla, turn off the heat and stir quickly to emulsify and melt the chocolate.

3. Pour the hot frosting over the brownies. It will cool fairly quickly, so do not pause between melting the chocolate and spreading the frosting. Pick up the brownie pan and roll the frosting over the entire top. If you're topping with walnuts, sprinkle them on now.

4. Once cooled, cut into 12 pieces. These brownies freeze well when individually wrapped in plastic.

What was great about working at CCC was being able to be creative and experiment with food with other people that love food. I've never worked anywhere else that gave you chocolate, mushroom powder, and sour cherries, and said go ahead, make a delicious dessert.
- Ryan Lucas (baker)

gluten-free & vegan brownies

SAVANNAH VILLA **1 HOUR & 30 MINUTES** **YIELDS 12 BROWNIES**   **GLUTEN-FREE**   **VEGAN**

Savannah's recipe makes a particularly beautiful brownie with its lace of ganache and button-like dots of chocolate chip puckering its thin crispy top. You can use your favorite gluten-free flour mix or try our easy-to-make Oat Flour Dry Mix. Oat flour creates a fibrous texture, which gives the brownie good "tooth", or chewiness.

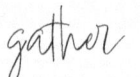   **mixing bowl, measuring cups, measuring spoons, rubber spatula, 9 x 13-inch pan**

BROWNIES

2 cups white sugar

¾ cup cocoa powder
(Hershey's)

¾ tsp baking powder

¾ tsp baking soda

1 tsp kosher salt

2 ½ cups Oat Flour Dry Mix, recipe follows *sub any g.f. flour mix

1 cup canola oil

1 ½ tsp vanilla extract

1 cup vegan chocolate chips, divided

1 cup hot drip coffee

vegan pan spray

1. Heat the oven to 350°.

2. Mix the sugar, cocoa powder, baking powder, baking soda, kosher salt, and Oat Flour Dry Mix in a mixing bowl.

3. Add the canola oil, vanilla extract, and ¾ cup chocolate chips. Melt the chocolate chips by pouring in the hot coffee. Fold together, being careful not to over-mix.

4. Coat the baking pan with the pan spray, then pour in the batter. Use the spatula to even out the batter in the pan. Sprinkle the remaining ¼ cup of chocolate chips on top of the batter.

5. Bake for 35-40 minutes. Test with the toothpick method. Let cool for 20 minutes.

VEGAN GANACHE

½ cup vegan chocolate chips

6 Tbsp coconut milk, canned

1. Melt the vegan chocolate chips and coconut milk in a microwave for approx. 1 ½ minutes or until the chocolate has melted. Whisk together. You can also use the double boil method.

2. Drizzle the ganache over the brownies in a cross-hatch pattern. Cool, then cut into 12 even pieces. These brownies freeze well when individually wrapped in plastic.

pro tip

Double boil method - Boil 2 cups of water in a small pot. Place a metal mixing bowl on top of the pot containing the chocolate chips (and any additional ingredients). As the water boils, the chocolate will melt. Use a whisk or fork to mix them together.

OAT FLOUR DRY MIX

1 cup oat flour, sifted

¾ cup white rice flour

¼ cup brown rice flour

¼ cup + 2 Tbsp tapioca starch

1 Tbsp + 1 ½ tsp white sugar

1 ¾ tsp xanthum gum

½ tsp iodized salt

½ tsp cream of tartar

1. Mix all ingredients together. Note: If you cannot find oat flour in the grocery store, spin oats in a blender until their texture is nearly dust. If you still have chunks, sift, and re-blend.

acknowledgments

This book was a community-supported project. Owners Barb and Carla, current and ex-employees, friends of the restaurant, and my personal community, all stepped up to help me create this cookbook. The endeavor spanned almost two years and regularly tested my resilience as I bumped against the limits of my knowledge, skills, and experience. There were moments when I almost threw down my towel and walked off the line. Inevitably, someone would come along and tell me how important it was to record this bit of the Cafe's history, or how they couldn't wait to cook a Cafe favorite at home. I'd clean off my station and get back to work. The cookbook didn't feel real until I received the first draft of the recipe format from prep cook/graphic designer, Chelsea Bobula. When I saw server/artist, Melissa Weisser's, painting of the Cafe, which now graces the cookbook's cover, I was in tears as I grasped the importance of documenting this amazing group of people, the owners, and the food we created together. Many heartfelt thanks are due.

Carla Blumberg and Barb Neubert - The biggest thanks go out to you for creating this visionary space. Thank you for trusting me to run your restaurant and to honor it by writing this cookbook. Without your blessing and continued support, this book would have never happened. Carla - Your brilliance and clear vision for the big picture has been a steady inspiration. Thank you for trusting me to write this cookbook. You are a role model and mentor to me both in the kitchen and out. Barb - You taught me lessons that I will always hold dear: to have integrity, to hold myself and others accountable for their actions, and that blunt honesty is a great tool. Your standards became the little voice in my head that informed my decisions about the restaurant and this book. Danielle

Sosin - Your professional advice was a goddess-send when I needed help. Thank you for being available for my endless questions, for making sense of and shaping my words. You helped me find my voice, the point of the story, and the point of this entire project. This book would be a jumbled mess without you. Chelsea Bobula - There are too many things to thank you for, from cheerleading to photos, to design and layout, to working with my ever-changeable mind. You were a driver of this project. It really couldn't have happened without you.

To the recipe contributors - Your hard work, culinary talent, and creativity have made the restaurant memorable, and this book fantastic! The spotlight should really be on you: Peter Ravinski, Bruce Wallis, Natalie Allesee, Avery Cassar, Diane Bailey, Carla Blumberg, Barb Neubert, Heather Erickson, Rita Bergstedt, Jeremy Barany, Colleen Betts, Kirsten Aune, Matt Lindberg, Lyndon Ramrattan.

To the incredibly talented illustrators - Thank you for bringing your vision to my incomplete ideas. You put the pictures to my thoughts: Emily Koch, Melissa Weisser, Cristina Plascencia, Benjamin Zaban-Boylan, Amanda Clark.

Thank you recipe testers - You gave me invaluable feedback (and let me know that my prep times were way too short for the average cook!) Sarah, Josh, Brita & Odin Carlson, Anthony Fiorillo, Elizabeth Johnson, Ellen Vaagen, Lisa Radosevich-Craig, Zora Radosevich, Dan Monson, Hans Bjorklund, Julie Louise Koski, Mary Bue, Cynthia Joe, Tajen Stockdale, Kathy Radosevich, Lisa Luokkala, Lane Johnson, Leona Luokkala-Schmidt.

Gratitude to all my coworkers who contributed "Tips and Tricks" to these pages. Home cooks will significantly benefit from your experience and words of advice: Heather Erickson, Rachel Anvary, Colleen Betts, Ben Butter, Channie McCall, Brandon Helberg, Casey Watsula, Sterling Smythe, Jackie Fontaine, Lino Rauzi, Tony Bosak, Kirsten Aune, Hana Gaudreau, Savannah Villa, Christopher Sheppard, Katie Schmitz.

To everyone I interviewed, or who sent me a Cafe story. We giggled, snickered, and teared up. Memory lane was so sweet to share with you: Sonja Helland, Faith Woodruff, AJ Choi, Rolf Holvik, Jackie Fontaine,

Sarah Maxim, Carey Kasapidis, Peter Ravinski, Jenny (Plitcher) Quinn, Shelly Barry, Kelly Rubel, Jesse Erickson, Ben Hoffmeister, Ryan Lucas, Anna Brown, Jesse Hoheisel, Dave Rogotski, Lynda and Lee Dietrich, Colleen Betts, Heather Erickson, Peter Ravinski, Diane Bailey, Amy Nakamura, Rita Bergstedt, Shaunna Heckman, Tony Bosak & Max Moen.

And to everyone else who helped me along the way technically and emotionally! You were there when I needed you: Amy Kozak, Matt Lindberg, Chris Forte, Ramiro Figueroa, Rigail Cumbe, Emily Ostos, Shari Bradt, Samantha Kabourek, Sharla Gardner, Jessica Skarman, Molly Lamphear.

Special thanks to my rock, Rocco Salvatore, my parents Bob and Linda Forte, and my kiddo Aurora. Last but not least, thank you to my Abuelita Manuela Forte for being the one to show me the magic and joy of cooking for loved ones.

index

INDEX BY CHEF

ILLUSTRATORS

gluten-free

10,000 Lakes Dressing 138

Award-Winning Rhubarb Chutney 118

Baja Slaw 67

Bloody Mary Mix 50

Blue Cheese Dressing 137

Breakfast Sausage 49

Bright Green BasilPesto 105

Cabernet Braised Beef 75

Caramelized Onions 61

Carrot Ginger & Quinoa Soup 153

Chester Creek Tomato Bisque 147

Chevre Potato Tarts 113

Classic Hummus 60

Coconut Cauliflower "Rice" 77

Colorful Baja Fish Tacos 67

Compound Butter 100

Cranberry Peach Chutney 117

Crispy Polenta 76

Curried Winter Squash Soup 155

Delicata, Pickled Beets & Herbed Goat Cheese
    Salad with Mustard Vinaigrette 127

Fish Taco Seasoning 67

Garlic Chili Sauce 86

Gluten-Free & Vegan Brownies 171

Gluten-Free Pancakes 45

Golden Gohbi Matar Soup 151

Golden Rice 97

Green Buddha Bowl 83

Grilled Jerk Chicken 78

Hard Boiled Eggs 122

Harissa Aioli 107

Hippie Farm 37

Honey Mustard 62

Kung Fu Noodle Bowl 63

Lamb Kefta Kabobs 79

Lemon-Dijon Vinaigrette 129

Lime Caper Aioli 66

Malbec Vinaigrette 125

Maple Mascarpone 47

Maple-Sherry Vinaigrette 133

Massaged Kale Salad * with G.F. Tamari 136

Matt's Kimchi 109

Mexican Caldo de Res 152

Moroccan Chicken Tagine & Couscous 87

Okonomiyaki 53

Original Thai Curry - Chicken or Tofu 91

Pickled Beets 127

Pico de Gallo 106

Pimento Cheese Spread 116

Poached Eggs 130

Pork Pho Noodle Bowl 159

Potato Parsnip Puree 111

Quinoa Veggie Burger 57

Ras el Hanout 87

Raspberry Vinaigrette 139

Saffron Sofrito 98

Seared Brussels Sprouts 112

Shrimp, Scallops & Chorizo Paella 97

Smoked Salmon Seasoning 119

Spicy Vegan Aioli 55

Spinach, Feta & Tomato Breakfast Salad
    with Goddess Dressing 135

Tahini Sauce 84

Thai Chicken Coconut Soup 149

Tofu & Tempeh (T&T) Marinade 121

Tzatziki 79

Vietnamese Braised Beef Short Ribs 85

Wild Rice Risotto 100

Yucatan Carnitas Tacos 69

GLUTEN-FREE WITH SUBSTITUTIONS

Asparagus & Poached Egg Salad with
    Lemon-Dijon Vinaigrette 129

Beef Bulgogi Tacos 70

Deluxe Grilled Cheese 64

Grilled Steak , Asparagus & Mushroom
    Salad with Malbec Vinaigrette 125

Ham & Gouda Melt, Honey Mustard &
    Caramelized Onions 61

Marathon Meatballs 93

Minnesota Wild Rice, White Fish & Roasted
    Root Vegetables 99

Roasted Corn Poblano Chowder 154

Root Vegetable Panzanella with Maple-
    Sherry Vinaigrette 131

Rosemary Cream & Butternut Squash Pasta 95

Vegan Bulgogi Tacos 71

vegetarian

VEGETARIAN WITH SUBSTITUTIONS OR OMISSIONS

vegan

VEGAN WITH SUBSTITUTIONS OR OMISSIONS

dairy-free

10,000 Lakes Dressing 138

Arroz Verde 115

Award-Winning Rhubarb Chutney 118

Beef Bulgogi Tacos 70

Beef Stock 146

Bloody Mary Mix 50

Breakfast Sausage 49

Cabernet Braised Beef 75

Caramelized Onions 61

Carrot, Ginger & Quinoa Soup 153

Chicken Stock 145

Classic Hummus 60

Coconut Cauliflower "Rice" 77

Colorful Baja Fish Tacos 67

Cranberry Peach Chutney 117

Garlic Chili Sauce 86

Gluten-Free & Vegan Brownies 171

Gluten-Free Pancakes 45

Goddess Dressing 135

Golden Gohbi Matar Soup 151

Golden Rice 97

Green Buddha Bowl 83

Grilled Jerk Chicken 78

Harissa Aioli 107

Kirsten's Hard Boiled Egg 122

Kung Fu Noodle Bowl 63

Lamb Kefta Kabobs 81

Lemon Dijon Vinaigrette 129

Lemony Tabbouleh 59

Lime Caper Aioli 66

Maple-Sherry Vinaigrette 133

Massaged Kale Salad 136

Matt's Kimchi 109

Mexican Caldo de Res 152

Morning Glory Muffins 163

Moroccan Chicken Tagine & Couscous 87

Oat Flour Dry Mix 172

Oatmeal Stout Beer Syrup 48

Okonomiyaki 53

Original Thai Curry - Chicken or Tofu 91

Pico de Gallo 106

Pork Pho Noodle Bowl 159

Quinoa Veggie Burger 57

Ras el Hanout 87

Raspberry Vinaigrette 139

Roasted Root Vegetables 99, 132

Seafood Burger 65

Seared Brussels Sprouts 112

Shrimp, Scallop & Chorizo Paella 97

Smoked Salmon Seasoning 119

Spicy Vegan Aioli 55

Tahini Sauce 84

Thai Chicken Coconut Soup 149

Tofu & Tempeh (T&T) Marinade 121

Vegan Bulgogi Tacos 71

Vegetable Stock 144

Veggie Loaded Beef Stew 157

Vietnamese Braised Beef Short Ribs & Garlic Chili Sauce 85

Yucatan Carnitas Tacos 69

DAIRY-FREE WITH SUBSTITUTIONS OR OMISSIONS

Asparagus & Poached Egg Salad with Lemon-Dijon Vinaigrette 129

Chester Creek Tomato Bisque 147

Curried Winter Squash Soup 155

Delicata, Pickled Beets & Herbed Goat Cheese Salad with Mustard Vinaigrette 127

Golden Gohbi Matar Soup 151

Grilled Steak, Asparagus & Mushroom Salad with Malbec Vinaigrette 125

Hippie Farm 37

Marathon Meatballs 93

Roasted Corn Poblano Chowder 154

Root Vegetable Panzanella with Maple-Sherry Vinaigrette 133

Spinach, Feta, Tomato Breakfast Salad with Goddess Dressing 135

Spinach, Feta & Tomato Breakfast Salad with Goddess Dressing 135

keto

KETO WITH SUBSTITUTIONS OR OMISSIONS